THE CLIFFS OF SCHIZOPHRENIA

A MOTHER AND SON PERSPECTIVE

A Memoir

JAKE & LAURETTE McCOOK

The Cliffs of Schizophrenia
Jake & Laurette McCook

Print ISBN 979-8-35092-596-8
eBook ISBN 979-8-35092-597-5

"I'm standing on the edge of some crazy cliff. What I have to do, I have to catch everybody if they start to go over the cliff, I mean if they're running and they don't look where they're going, I have to come out from somewhere and catch them. That's all I do all day. I'd just be the catcher in the rye and all. I know it's crazy, but that's the only thing I'd really like to be."

—J. D. Salinger, *The Catcher in the Rye*

CONTENTS

THE DISORDER
Jake

You stop everything to decode yourself.

The world stops for you to slow down.

Everyone is polite. Everyone is still.

You break yourself down until there is nothing left,

Until nothing makes sense.

You are exhausted. You are cornered.

Everyone holds back their frayed emotions as they play

verbal ping-pong with you for the thousandth time.

You are angry. You are empathetic.

You love them, and they love you.

Their lies are the foundation of your truth, the building blocks

of your stunted emotions.

UNTETHERED

Mom

His clean-shaven face radiates the ragged goodness of a ten-year-old boy, but late afternoon light flickers its epiphany of manhood, and my eyes sting with all that is lost. Purity of baby skin and clear-eyed innocence, a subterranean beast to haunt my days and nights.

Messages on trucks and T-shirts and the Nightly News, a searing reality of delusion that perches uneasily upon a fragile surface. His face gazing back at me through staircase railing as he sits silently seeking answers to riddles no mother should have to answer.

Silent and useless, there is palpable pain that runs like umbilical cord between us wearily pumping a haunting refrain of maternal promises unfulfilled. Earthbound, while he soars to places, I cannot follow. Sweet eyes that linger a moment, then are gone.

Clarity is hope and hope is . . . what?

TO THE READER
Jake

I want this book to be a safe haven for you, a place to be open and honest about your own issues with schizophrenia. Find a cozy spot, sit with your worries, and let this book swallow them up and temporarily rid you of them. A transference. A swapping of stories for stories. I'll take yours in my hands and hold them for a short while, as you read mine. I hope this will give you some relief.

THE CLIFFS OF

SCHIZOPHRENIA

A MOTHER AND SON PERSPECTIVE

INTRODUCTION
Mom

"Are dinosaurs real?" My twenty-eight-year-old son appeared in the room where I was folding laundry. He drew in a labored breath. It seemed as though he might spontaneously combust right there in front of me, so his tight exhale came as a relief for both of us.

"Hey, kiddo, what a nice surprise. What's up?" His visit was unexpected, as it was only mid-day and he'd not been home much since the move to his new apartment in Burbank the previous month. Something felt amiss. His lanky frame stooped forward; his hands jammed into his pockets.

"The dinosaurs . . . I mean, I'm not sure," he whispered, his eyes darted right to see if anyone else was in the room.

Instinct slowed me. "Sure, honey, they're . . . they were very real." He didn't speak then, so I continued. "Right? I mean you've seen so many cartoons and Jurassic Park type movies; it's probably easy to forget that you learned about dinosaurs in school." I watched him draw in another breath while nodding his head. He turned away from me and clicked on the television. The moment passed quickly.

I have no recollection of how I processed that. I guess I didn't. A door had slammed shut in my head, and I simply blocked the dark thing that had announced its presence as a mere flicker of fear on my son's face. Those early years were filled with bits and pieces of abstract information that would come and go. It was a clue that tweaked my logic and yet . . . I had to let it go.

Looking back, twelve years is a long road—an information overload on a journey both terrifying and bewildering, but as in any crisis, life comes at you one day at a time so as not to break you all at once. It took years for Jake to be properly diagnosed and medicated. Schizophrenia is a brain disease. It has taken so much from all of us, and recently it occurred to me that writing a book might be the answer. He'd always had a way with words and of uniquely expressing his ideas . . . but could he stay focused on a project these days, long enough to see it through? And could dredging up the past open the Pandora's box of paranoia that dogs Jake every moment of the day and night? This book was his idea, the concept of schizophrenia from a family perspective, a journal moving back and forth between mother and son. He felt it should be written in brief chapters so as not to overwhelm a reader who has symptoms like his. This would be a comfort food for those lonely moments when you feel different from everyone else on the planet.

The writing process was cathartic for Jake, as well as disruptive, in that reliving his experiences did indeed kick off some pretty substantial waves of depression and paranoia.

Nevertheless, he persevered, saying that he wanted and needed to keep writing to get his story out there. It is this bravery I am in awe of every day.

During the time it took to finish this book, all of us have gone through a great deal: political unrest, a worldwide pandemic, and environmental chaos. To the average person, we are shaken . . . but for those with mental illness, it is a minefield of triggers to the dark side. With so much yet unanswered in the quest to find peace in a brain that is at war within itself, we journey on together ever seeking the path that will bring mental illness out of the dark ages and into the light. Oh, we're waking up, and it's in vogue to make statements on social media declaring allegiance, but we're searching with a flashlight. If you or a loved one is experiencing this battle, then you are well aware what we are up against, and it is a lonely and scary war indeed. This book is for Jake and for you.

IN THE BEGINNING

Jake

Everything that occurred prior to the onset of schizophrenia was perfect. A dream. A vanilla sky of creation. Since I was nine years old and on into my twenties, before there were YouTube careers and Instagram advertising partners, I was churning out videos by the hundreds in hopes of getting a laugh from my parents, sisters, or friends.

I had a solid troupe of actors at my disposal. Mainly my family. My youngest sister, Molly, was the Meryl Streep of the bunch. She was passionate, devoted, and able to take direction like nobody's business. Today, she's a successful television actress. My sister Becky took a little more arm twisting to be in a video, but she was always hilarious. These days she's a television producer.

One of the best McCook movies was *Grandma Baba*. Molly wore an old man mask with a wig and a prim dress and wreaked havoc on her grandkid's social life with constant flatulence and raiding of the family fridge. One cannot forget the unsettling trilogy I made with my best buddy "Stomachache" where two friends binge eat and then vomit on screen for an uncomfortable amount of time.

These were the bookmarks of my emotional life. If I was frustrated with my social life, I would make a movie about twins that worked out their relationship issues on a split screen. If I needed to exorcise my demons, I would make a music video and spastically dance or wildly lip sync to some current pop song.

It was what I needed. It was my drug of choice, and I couldn't stop. I was hooked. Maybe it was being able to control people. All of it. My true friends were a video camera, a computer, and a jumble of studio lights. It was insulation that protected me from the outside world—the distraction from an adult life that would one day steal my joy, my independence, and my dreams of a world where anything was possible.

FOR PARENTS
Mom

When did I know that my son had a mental illness? Hindsight unearths little red flags that lie just beneath the surface of his childhood. But can you really know what's ahead, and are there markers you should watch out for?

Perhaps my first flickering of a problem that barely registered at my core was during nursery school when the school director called us with a concern regarding Jake's tendency to play alone. He would be so focused on his toys, she said, that he blocked out everything else. "So what," I asked? "A child can't be focused?" We were angry that she suggested medication might be the answer. He was four, for Lord's sake. How dare she! Right?

The years going forward had plenty of kid-type drama but nothing concerning or abnormal. His grades were fine. He excelled in vocabulary and creative writing. Math and foreign language were not his thing. Nor mine, as I recall. By fourth grade, he was lucky enough to have a sharp teacher, who midway through the year, suggested we have him tested. He ranked high in visual perception, writing, and really all things that would soon lead him to his lifetime love of film and editing. Now and then, I found myself using the term, "falling between the cracks" when describing Jake's gifts as well as his learning abilities. It was obvious to all that he was highly creative, and he had his own special way about him. We were always proud of that.

Social interaction was sometimes an issue, but this is where it got confusing. Kids in his class loved him and included him. He was shy and very kind. We were amused by his need for order in school and home. If the family was going somewhere together, Jake always needed to know exactly where his sisters were and if parents and grandma were all accounted for. We got used to reassuring him. It's still that way.

When did I know my son had a problem? The answer is that I didn't. It is only now that I can go back, in hindsight, when one is suddenly omniscient. How can a mother or father know absolutely that their child will one day be mentally ill? Who among us can pinpoint the moment as it happens because it is never one moment. It is a collection of moments . . . an entire childhood and then some, until some doctor shatters your world with the words, "Your son has schizophrenia." There were many diagnoses before we came to that road, and they all left us feeling terrified in the pit of our stomachs. But I have never ever given up. You will be told to "accept." That took me years. But within my acceptance is a hope that will never go away. A better life for him. Together we will find the best possible life that he can manage . . . and so will you.

Acceptance will help you keep your parental sanity. Hope will be your driving force.

MOVIE MAKING FOR THE SOUL
Jake

Movie making was everything to me. At thirteen, I got a Panasonic WJ MX-12 Video Mixer for my birthday, which at the time was as cool as getting Final Cut Pro X today. It mixed music, provided shape video transitions, and allowed me to hook up to as many as four VCRs. I had a friend whose dad was a TV movie director. He knew I wanted to be an editor and gave me ten or so VHS dailies from one of his films. It helped shape my style as I practiced cutting scenes together.

In seventh grade, my school entered the class in a mock trial competition. We were assigned roles as lawyers, bailiffs, and witnesses. I was so terrified of performing in front of people that I went to my teacher and cried. Luckily, she was a wonderful, empathetic person. "Why don't you film the whole experience for us?" Yes!

I started mapping out the soundtrack in my mind. "Nick of Time" and "Sudden Death" were excellent thriller movie scores. Creating a video for my class was a fantasy of mine.

It would be my way of trading my video for their friendship; I did have a small group of friends but wanted to be accepted by everyone.

I was able to film the class from a distance and even had a moment with a girl that I liked, chasing her down with my camera, hoping to have a smart conversation with her using my camera armor to protect me from social harm. Of course, she giggled and ran in the opposite direction.

We ended up in second place, and I premiered the video in front of all the kids in my class. I got a huge round of applause and finally felt I belonged.

By fifteen, I was inserting myself into movie trailers. I had done it pretty well with *U.S. Marshals* and wanted to do it with *Crimson Tide*. I had figured a way to record shots of myself, then put them into movie previews so that the sound from the trailer carried over. I would take the raw trailer and tape over that, a chunk at a time with my camera footage.

It was a great time in my life. I could put on a white sports coat of my dad's and be Brad Pitt in *Fight Club*, with me mouthing Pitt's lines. Or even Denzel in *Crimson Tide* . . . which leads me to a stunt I wanted to pull off where Denzel was slammed against the wall of a submarine by Gene Hackman. I had to use what I could work with, which in my case was a glass shower door in my bathroom. I set up my camera and pushed "record," then hurled myself against the glass.

Not good enough. Take Two. It needed to be even harder. I wanted the sound of the door to be louder.

Take Three. I jumped this time, getting some air under my feet, then crashed against the door. The glass shattered on impact with ear-deafening noise. I must've blacked out for a second because I woke up sitting inside the shower with huge shards of glass on my lap. There was blood everywhere, and strangely, I felt no pain. Heart pounding, I edged myself out of the narrow space. My corduroy pants probably saved my life. I was immediately ecstatic that I'd gotten what I wanted from the stunt. I couldn't wait to show everyone.

Heading down the hallway of our house, I hoped to find my sisters. Our parents were out to dinner nearby. There was blood on my hands and shirt. Way cool. The girls were both in the playroom, and I yelled out to them. They popped up from the couch and turned toward me. At first, they didn't respond, just stared at me.

"Icutmyselfontheshowerdoor," Iannounceddramatically.

"Really?" Becky said sarcastically. Then she and four-year-old Molly walked up to me, suddenly uncertain as to whether I was really okay.

"You want to see the shower?" I blurted.

"Yeah . . . sure!" they both shouted back. We ran into the bathroom, and Becky surveyed the damage. It looked like a crime scene. "Oh my God," she whispered. "I think we need to call Mom and Dad."

Cut and print.

EXPRESSION OF THE SOUL
Mom

Jake made movies day and night. If his friends wanted to see him, then they had to come over to his house and be in one of his movies, which many of them did over the years. School kids, neighborhood kids, family friends, and relatives. My favorites were the jock kids. They clearly felt awkward acting, but he always lured them into a hitman scenario, military highjinks, or the ever popular gross out vomit movie. I had to keep my pantry stocked for those. Ketchup was at a premium.

We'd often let him have showings of his movies for his sisters and their friends. He and his best friend spent several years making movies. Looking back on those days, you'd think Jake was wildly uninhibited. When he was alone in his room with the cameras . . . or with his best buddy creating, he was a force to be reckoned with. As an actor, he was believable, smart, and very funny with a Jim Carrey sort of abandon. He wrote all his own material on many topics: the absurd, family life, film reviews, talk show take-offs, murder mysteries on location, and even an occasional serious topic like death, drugs (complete with a warning message), or current events. If his dad, sisters, and I wanted to spend time with Jake, we would just agree to be in one of his films. His Grandma Evie was always the good sport, to the extent that one time, she sat in a kitchen chair with her hands bound behind her back, butcher knife to her throat, and a large red apple clamped between her teeth. He got a time-out for that stunt.

Oh, and about that ill-fated *Crimson Tide* night; Jake's dad and I were five minutes away at a nearby restaurant. My phone rang, and our daughter Becky's voice sounded uneasy. "Jake fell through the shower door and there's blood everywhere." I don't know how we made it home safely.

His dad was both scared and angry with him that he'd been so careless. "Are you alright?" he asked gripping his shoulders, then, "How could you be so stupid?" Thank God, Jake was wearing long pants and sleeves, so the surface cuts were on his hands, wrists, and a few on his face. He was rosy with excitement and stopped his dad mid-sentence. "Dad . . . Dad . . . I GOT THE SHOT!!"

And so it was in Jake's world. Getting the shot was all that mattered. Later, we had to laugh . . . somewhat nervously, but there was pride that he gave his all. Now we had to teach him safety. It was brutal to have to watch the slow-motion replay that Jake proudly showed us over and over as he backed through a heavy glass door. I aged ten years that night.

High school became a challenge in many ways. He was a handsome and charming boy but still had that self-effacing way about him. His buddy Jonathon from next door was at the school dance that year, and Jake was awed by how easy it seemed for this boy to be the center of attention. He could take off his shirt and twirl it over his head, then make the girls laugh and focus only on him. How was that possible? Jake admired him a great deal, but then the boy also admired Jake because he knew what he wanted to be. A filmmaker. All the kids thought of Jake that way.

Today, as I work with my son on this book, I can clearly see one thing has not changed. Creativity is still Jake's center. Music, painting, sketching, video editing, and especially his ability to express the inexpressible in his writing. A beacon on the journey forward.

A TASTE FOR INSANITY

Jake

Somewhere around twenty-three years old, I actually remember thinking that it would be cool to be a bit of a recluse . . . and a touch crazy. I'd seen the actor Ed Harris in a wonderful film about Jackson Pollock. I read a biography about him and felt inspired and connected to the artist and what he stood for, which was organic, off-the-cuff creation.

He was able to create in a haze of alcoholism and what was then thought of as just plain crazy. He was later rumored to have been bipolar.

Just as Pollock inspired me as I got older, Jim Carrey was the lighthouse through my teens. My goal back then was to be as spastically funny as he was. Cut to twenty years later and I'm walking through a Jim Carrey art exhibit in downtown Los Angeles, a huge gallery filled with sketches he'd done in a very short period of time. They were socially and politically relevant while maintaining his sharp sense of humor. I was blown away. Here's a guy also rumored to be bipolar or certainly on the spectrum, and he's still hanging on to the same thread that I am.

Now that I look back at the Pollock days, I wonder if I was born mentally ill, and that my obsession with him was based solely on the fact that he was also mentally ill and an alcoholic who was successfully making a career for himself despite his illness.

ODE TO DEPAKOTE

Mom

What is that oft used Einstein quote about insanity? It's doing the same thing again and again, each time expecting different results.

Wait, that's me. I always begin each day hoping today is the day. Today, Jake will not wake up under that cloud of depression. He'll see and feel that life has more to offer him. He will taste hope and decide that he really does want to find that magical mix of medications that hold the promise of a better life for him. A balance of feeling and thought. At times, I stand on the periphery of his perfect storm of catastrophe that strips him of reason and reality, leaving him unable to recognize his own illness. Anosognosia. That's the term for "lack of insight." Jake hates that word. The big words don't help, do they?

Schizophrenia twists Jake's ability to fix himself. He cannot really understand that by staying the course . . . remaining sober and clean, he might find happiness. Of course, I can't promise him these things either, but I have reason to hope. A mother's hope.

So, his doctor prescribed Depakote a few weeks ago. What is Depakote? It's an anti-epileptic. It treats seizures from epilepsy or from a seizure Jake might have from all the medications he's taking. It treats manic symptoms in bipolar disorder. Most of these medications also have what I call an "oh, by the way" perk, something that creates improvement in an area other than what it was prescribed for. Many doctors prescribe it as a mood stabilizer as well as in treatment of migraines. Who knew?

It took many months for Jake to accept the last two medications he tried as it's a scary process for him. No matter how great the results are, it always depends on the time of day, the moment, the mood. If you are reading this book, then you already get it . . . that the person with this illness doesn't truly believe that meds are the answer, no matter what. In fact, even if I witness with my own eyes that Jake is having a good day, it is likely that his own take will be the opposite.

While my heart soars with a seemingly small improvement, Jake will express extreme trepidation and an almost cynical view of the med not working or that it is making him feel too clear or alert. This clarity is the good part for me, for it is the clarity that returns his brain to a more normal state of viewing the world, without the din of thoughts and fog of confusion.

In Jake's head, this clarity seems to push him forward so that the smallest social interaction feels like it's a violation. In your face!

Jake and I have these conversations over and over. I take on the voice of reason and calm, trying to convince him of all the good things I see in him on this medication. He listens . . . patiently . . . or I think he does, but there are really no words that can draw him into a reality that does not exist for him. I watch him taking in my words. I see that although he loves me and wants to please me, he does not . . . cannot grasp this reality being a good thing. He cannot put another pill into a body that he truly feels is dying. Is he being poisoned, he asks me. At this moment, even I am a suspect.

Do I feel frustrated? You have no idea. I can feel my heart beating hard in my chest. How can he not get it? It truly feels like we're speaking different languages. My heartbreak is that I hurt him every time I say things like, "My God, Jake, how can you NOT see this? Please trust me. I'm your mom!" On and on I go imparting wisdom wrapped in mother's arms, and my pleading continues as he slips more into what he feels is utter failure.

Four days on Depakote and I'm telling you he was almost without paranoia and anxiety. No panic attacks in four days. Everyone today casually uses the words "panic attack" as if a rough day of stressful events is all it is. In reality, it is a claustrophobic, sweating, drooling, heart-racing assault in which you are certain that your heart will stop in the next second, lips blue from lack of oxygen and you have seconds to live. Your body is shutting down. Your brain fills with despair, and this moment is unstoppable. THAT is a real panic attack. Nothing less. I have not had one, but I've witnessed many. It's brutal to watch your child in pain and know that it's inside his head, a place I cannot reach.

Am I at peace with encouraging him to take these pills all the time? Of course not. I want him to feel happy and whole without having to take something. BUT this illness will not allow him to have that! If you're diabetic, you might be required to take insulin. Cancer points to radiation, medication, or chemo. It is what you must do to balance yourself. To find your center and make it stable.

So, at the end of the four days on Depakote, things began to fall apart. He lost sight of how he felt, and questions arose. He skipped one day, then two. He felt worse, and ultimately paranoia swept back in and alcohol was the only thing to stop the sudden onslaught of bad thoughts.

This week is all about recovery. Getting back on track and trying to trust each other again. I don't have the luxury of getting angry at him so that he'll realize his mistake and everything will make sense. We rebuild. Very slowly. His dad, Jake, and I slow it all down and reframe the battle that we're all in together.

Today, he has a new prescription to try. No more Depakote. A different mood stabilizer. This one is Topamax, a low dose. But it looms large in his daily pillbox. It's new and unknown. It has promise of great things for him. For Jake, it is loaded with uncertainty.

TOPAMAX

Jake

Here I sit. Staring at a tiny white pill. The size of the pupil in my eye. And it scares the shit out of me. Another anti-seizure med. I've been taking pills for too many years now. Two different antipsychotics plus anti-anxiety medication. Hard to remember sometimes as it changes so often. I've taken them easily these past months, so why should this new pill be any different? I'm afraid it will take me over the edge . . . over to death. It's been in my body two days already, so that's been done. I'm not sure if it's responsible for fewer panic attacks, but if I could be certain . . . I'd gladly take it.

There's just no way to know if it truly works. I didn't take it yesterday. I just pocketed it and went to sleep. Two borderline panic attacks followed, but I still can't be sure that it was only because I skipped the Topamax. My theory about panic attacks stemming from eating too much and too fast is almost proven . . . in my own head anyway.

Last night, I wanted to binge eat in the worst way, so I found myself hovering over Cheetos and Blue Diamond Almonds. I had once again forgotten the rule to not over-eat or I'd find myself in a panic. I was shoving food down my throat faster than I ever had. Thirty minutes later, I was shaking and pacing back and forth, desperately trying to find a solution. Luckily, it was minor this time, and I quickly took my nighttime meds early.

I had one of my lucid dreams about death that night. Drowning in some kind of liquid. Fighting for consciousness until I once again found myself on the side of the living . . . waking up grateful that I was still breathing but not sure how I could get through another day. That morning, I dragged my feet out of bed and placed them on solid ground. Daytime was the easy part. Who knew what another night would bring.

POCKETING PILLS
Mom

Too many pills have been in your life, my Jake. And none of them are your choice. Like me, you have always been lightweight when it comes to any medicines, so how is it that the past twelve years of your life has seen you on and off dozens of anti-depressant, anti-seizure, and anti-psychotic pills! It's just not right . . . or fair. I hate it too. But . . . these pills keep your brain quiet.

I want to remind you, Topamax is in the anti-seizure category. It protects you from having a full-blown seizure because of one of your other medications. Yeah, I know, stupid, right? But necessary and safer.

This said, I need to also remind you that pocketing or skipping pills just makes it worse. So take a deep breath and know that you're not alone in this journey. I'm reading labels, information, and picking the brain of every doctor we see. You will never be alone in this.

I LOVE MY FAMILY

Jake

It's incredible how panic can sneak up on you. One minute you're doing fine, talking with people, enjoying yourself, then in an instant, your eyes are darting around and trying to make sense of what each person is saying. Are they talking about you? Are they sending you a message?

Tonight, I was with my sister Becky, feeling good and not getting any bad vibes from her. All of a sudden, I had a need to express my discomfort with what I was saying, so I asked her if anything I was saying to her was offensive or hurtful. She immediately said no, and then told me if there was anything offensive, she would most certainly let me know. "Hey, bro," she said, she would say, "Hey, dude. What's up with that?"

On the tail of that, I caught wind of her husband Michel's conversation across the dinner table (don't get me started on dinner table crosstalk), and he was saying something about his parents. On hearing that, I jumped on the topic and decided to talk to Becky about Michel's parents too. "I had a conversation with Michel's dad on his last visit here," I said, ". . . and he's a nice guy." I don't know why I felt the need to do that. Looking for safety?

Becky agreed and said that they were living in Florida. I'd completely blown the mood with my paranoid bit, so I decided to get up and leave. "I'll talk to you later," I said, then rose and left the room as quickly as I could.

The second I got up, I worried that I'd bailed on our moment together in a weird and hurtful way. This is how you can corrupt a conversation by awkwardly departing. I wondered for a moment **why** it seemed so strange talking about Michel's parents. Nothing came to mind. I felt a bizarre sense of impending doom, as I couldn't understand why the moment had gone awry.

Suddenly, the rest of the family came rushing into the kitchen, or it sure seemed that way. I was now talking to my mom about all of it. I was waiting for an onslaught of words defending my sister and brother-in-law, but all I could hear were pieces of conversation around me. One from Michel; "I'm sorry," he said randomly.

Sorry? Sorry for what? This wasn't going to turn out well. The din quieted and once again . . . I left the room. Left the house. And soon the neighborhood. I made a beeline for the office where I pour out my soul for this book. After an hour of solitude, I feel almost 100 percent better. Yet, I know well that those thoughts will be waiting for me at home. For now, I averted a panic attack . . . and for that I am proud.

AND YOUR FAMILY LOVES YOU TOO!
Mom

I saw you closing off bit by bit during the day. It's been a really productive and positive two weeks, so today was a blip on the radar. You have close loving relationships with everyone in your family . . . except when we're all together in a group. That's it. Groups of people bring on confusion for you, and almost always incidents of crosstalk can send you into a tailspin. The misperception of information. Too many voices producing white noise in your head.

You left the house, and I was happy thinking of you at the office writing, although I was concerned about you being there after dark, thinking it might throw you off your game as you often react to change in mood and surroundings. You called my cell with great concern. I could hear it in your voice. "I'm feeling really weird. Like it's happening again."

My job at these moments is to be your grounding source. Steady and sure. "You're fine," I spoke quietly. "You've been good today. We all understand and support you." I went on to assure you that you had said nothing in the least offensive to anyone. You never do, although you believe otherwise. I wish I could convince you that your kindness and sensitivity is ever present.

I protect you too much. I don't entertain as often or easily as I'd like so that you don't have to be exposed to extra stress in your home. But I'm beginning to realize that you must be around people more often so that you can desensitize yourself to that crippling social anxiety. It's the one place that you are vulnerable.

You are loved and valued by each and every person in your family, Jake. No one blames you for this challenge you've been handed. If you want a visual, then picture us in a line of old, covered wagons. You are in the lead, and something up ahead scares you . . . your wagon abruptly stops. Slowly, the line of family in these other wagons begin to move past you, then around you, forming a circle . . . with you in the center. We're there to protect you. We've got your back, and you are never alone in this. Another mom-metaphor or mom-o-phor to quell the darkness.

SELF-MEDICATING
Jake

I can remember the first time I drank. It was with a friend who needed someone to drink with. I was about seventeen or eighteen, and he always had Canadian whiskey from his dad's stash. We would sit and watch porn while taking small gulps from the whiskey bottle. Occasionally, I would gag and not be able to take it in, but mostly I succeeded in building up my tolerance, which gave me a masculine pride. Gulp, stop. Gulp, gulp. Stop, gulp, gulp, gulp. Stop. I wasn't old enough to buy liquor, so I'd wait for my times with Canadian whiskey and my friend.

By the time I was twenty-one, I was a pro at hitting the liquor stores. I would always get Southern Comfort because it was simply . . . a comfort. Made those early thoughts and anxieties quiet down.

This is when I started stashing empty bottles in my dresser drawers. I had graduated from keeping down a little whiskey to finishing Southern Comfort bottles in two days. It was

the beginning of finding peace for my brain in any way that
I could.

MEDS AND BOOZE
Mom

There are times when I feel there's something wrong with me or the way I've chosen to handle my son's drinking or even his abuse of stimulant medications. For Jake, the stimulants are always a problem because they give him a quick surge of solid focus and reality that he desperately needs. These are powerful drugs, even in small doses. The emotional flatness or "blunting" that doctors observed later as a part of his illness was momentarily held at bay. Clarity and energy came with this one little pill. While the antidepressants and later the antipsychotics would do the core work, dealing with the depression, paranoia, and occasional delusions . . . the added stimulants like Adderall seemed to bring him to life. Remember, this is an amphetamine. I would soon lose sight of that.

My God, the day he met his dad and me for lunch in Sherman Oaks at a small outdoor cafe, he was newly on Adderall. A low but effective dose, or so we thought then. He walked up to our table with a wide smile, eyes bright and eager to talk. I almost cried. Here he was, back to his old self and much improved at that.

I know it sounds crazy, because you'd think we'd want that, to counter the meds that flattened him and left him groggy and without energy. If only it ended there. In a matter of weeks, we realized he was loving it a little too much. He had secretly increased his dose again and again. Jake was not yet on antipsychotics. Only Lexapro for depression. He soon announced he was out of his Adderall and needed more.

"What . . . already?" I asked. Within weeks, he was behaving oddly and acting paranoid, which I hadn't experienced in him before. He had panic attacks and told us that he thought he was being poisoned. We took him to the ER where I allowed him to use my cellphone to call his psychiatrist at UCLA. To my horror, Jake asked the doctor if he'd given him something to kill him. Well, not so much asked as accused. The doctor told me to stop the Adderall immediately. I couldn't figure out how he had gotten enough medication to increase it like that. Apparently, he'd saved it up . . . missing days in the beginning so that I'd never notice. I soon learned to count all meds as well as putting everything remotely buzz-worthy in a combination lockbox. Cold pills were gold. He'd taken three of my prescription migraine pills. Alcohol, and now pills? It seemed almost unimaginable that Jake would have this battle to wage, on top of what was going on in his brain.

Sometime during that year, Jake had an incident with a close friend who pranked him by leaving a bizarre helium-voiced message on his phone saying that he would kill him and "gut him like a pig," which I later learned was a line from the film Scream that they happened to have seen together. His buddy had no way of knowing that this message would launch Jake on his journey into mental illness. A highly traumatic moment. We had no idea who had done it as the voice was so altered. We reported it to the police. Jake told his friend what had happened, and he quickly confessed that he'd meant no harm. The ill-thought-out joke was sorted between the families, but the police insisted on following through with a visit. A scary time for both kids. This boy was like a member of our family, and we still love him dearly. Jake's break would have happened eventually anyway.

After that, the films he made began to change as some were tinged with paranoia; one in particular, was pure camera work. His bedroom . . . panning shot of the phone ringing, then slowly moving around a shadowed room in all directions. My sister, Marilyn, pointed out the darkness of the piece and wondered if the whole thing had been more disturbing than we realized.

Sadly, the boy's long friendship faded as Jake closed off more and more. He moved into an apartment in Burbank and went to work editing. He still made his personal films and took film classes, but there was little socializing after that. I imagine these were the prodromal signs. Drinking increased, and he found solace there.

Recently, Jake told me that it was the only way he could quiet his brain; otherwise, it was active 24/7. He once described his thoughts as a thousand Ping-Pong balls being shot in his direction. These thoughts often came in sets of three, and he would have to choose. Only one was correct. I cried myself to sleep that night. No matter how we tried to protect him, there would be no sheltering him from the constant assault going on inside his head.

FULL METAL JACKET
Jake

When I was twenty-three, I finally found a real industry job, video editing for a small but prestigious editing company. Their best work was producing A&E *Biography*, and they'd shot at least ten episodes, winning an Emmy for one. While I was there, Brian, the president of the company had a film he'd shot years ago with his wife who was a former child star. He admired my short films and wanted me to re-edit his wife's film into something more up-to-date and modern. He then filmed a psychologist explaining the effects of child stardom and interviews with his mother-in-law for me to splice in with the old footage.

This company president was odd, to say the least, and could have been diagnosed by a child . . . just by looking at him. He was a blurter and a bully. He said whatever came into his head. At one point, he got in my face, rolled his eyes back into his head, and snarled, "Full . . . Metal . . . Jacket." Then, "Give your parents my condolences." If you haven't seen the first half of *Full Metal Jacket*, it's about a mentally challenged marine who goes crazy and kills his drill instructor. I never considered myself to be mentally challenged, and least of all crazy. This moment would forever be stuck in my brain like a splinter. I was never able to remove it, though I tried.

At the time, I was living in Burbank, and every day after editing at work, I would come home to my apartment and focus on another project. I was burning the candle at both ends, and it wasn't good. My only social life was at work. I was taking Adderall, which is an attention deficit type of stimulant. I took it almost every day and abused it consistently.

On my computer at home, I had organized folders as well as I could. Movie Footage. Scripts. And then my most private stuff was in the folder marked "Cassie." A girl I met and hoped would be more.

One time while editing, my neighbors below me were talking loudly and I could make out words within sentences. I heard them say "Cassie" several times, then there was laughing. To me, the name Cassie, especially coupled with laughter, must have been because they were hacking into my computer. I became angry that someone was violating my privacy and decided to make a trip to my downstairs neighbor. I was sweating and shaking as I made my way to confront them. The voices from their apartment became louder as I approached their door. I took a moment to right myself, even though I knew this wasn't going to be easy. The door opened and the guy looked like he was in his early thirties and had a friendly air about him. I decided I'd just come out with it.

"Hi, my name is Jake and I live upstairs, directly above you. I overheard you talking about something that was on my computer."

"On your computer?"

"Yes, I have a folder on my desktop that says Cassie, and I've heard you say that name multiple times over the past half hour."

The neighbor looked at me like I was insane. "You think I'm hacking into your computer?"

"Yeah, I'm sorry . . . but yes, I think you are."

He looked behind him and shooed his young daughter away from the door. "Well, I'm sorry, Jake, but I'm not hacking into your computer."

"Are you sure?" I asked again.

"Yes, I'm positive." I apologized to him and slowly headed back upstairs, feeling like I needed to get outside and away from my apartment. I called my parents and told them I was coming home. I packed a few things and left. Once I got to their house, I lay down on the couch and tried to breathe. It was embarrassing knowing that I was the scary tenant upstairs. It was my first mental breakdown.

FIRST STEP INTO THE ABYSS
Mom

By Jake's early twenties, drinking was a part of his life. He kept his job in Burbank, but I soon learned that he was missing three to four days at a time. His boss made references at work to, "Jake going underground again." It cannot go unsaid that this man running the company was a horrible human being. He was verbally abusive to the young people who worked for him. Ridicule, profanity, and on one occasion throwing a coffee cup at Jake while a young secretary looked on weeping at her desk. I wish I'd known earlier than I did as there most certainly would have been a confrontation. In those days, all I knew was what Jake told me and that he was working at something he loved.

There were some good opportunities there and thankfully a few coworkers who were kind and caring. The stress continued, a toxic feeding ground for someone who is mentally ill. Jake's isolation grew. If I didn't hear from him for a few days, I called, texted, or ultimately drove to his apartment and rang the intercom on his building. When he didn't answer, I just sat on the front steps, scared and uncertain of what to do next. I left him messages from my cell, saying that I would not leave until he let me in. I'd sleep there if I must. At long last, I'd hear the intercom buzz behind me and bolt toward it, then straight up the stairs.

Jake's apartment was dark, with cigarette butts piled up over the edges of ashtrays, a few burns in the carpet, old food dried on plates that were stacked here and there on the coffee table, crumpled papers, dirty clothes, and his windows closed tight around a room that smelled of smoke and booze. He looked like he hadn't slept or bathed in days. He was nervous having me in his space and reluctant to talk, but we did. Or rather I did.

I've always been able to talk to Jake because I know his heart, and this is what hurt me. I could feel his fear and confusion. I couldn't tell if this was just plain old alcoholism, like so many in my family had faced. That made sense, but there was something more I couldn't place. Looking back, I believe I was too scared to think it.

His editing bay was set up in a small closet so that it jutted into the room. A pretty cool setup actually. This was sacred ground for Jake. His one connection to the real world. Then I noticed a sticky note covering the camera lens on his desktop computer. I asked him about it, and he waved me off. To this day, he has the camera covered on all his computers. I suppose it's not such a paranoid thought now to protect oneself from the rise in technology that comes into one's home, but when he was twenty-three, it was pure paranoia.

I cleaned his place in record time. I knew he might ask me to leave at any moment. I become supermom during cleanups because this is something I can do. Clean and give order to his environment, which ultimately helps him feel calm. I felt better leaving him this way, a picture of him standing in a nice apartment. A Band-Aid of sorts, but to this day, I find that Jake is always, always better in a well-organized surrounding.

Schizophrenia is disordered and chaotic. That day at the Burbank apartment was the beginning. We would all be living off the rails from here out. A clean apartment was literally the best I could do.

LUCID DREAMING
Jake

Last Saturday, I was in the middle of a lucid dream. I wish I could remember the details, but all I can recall is the moment I woke up. Still in the dream, I was walking outdoors and saw the face of a stranger. Suddenly, there was the sensation of my head dropping down and my mind failing in the matter of a second. The lucidity of the dream helped me fight what seemed to be happening to me.

I woke in my bed, fighting for consciousness, forcing myself to speak but only mumbling gibberish. By some miracle, I ended up on the side of the living. I took a deep breath and opened my eyes. I have been having this type of lucid dream for months and always around the same time. Five or six in the morning. This one was the worst and the most visceral. I'm lucky I'm not dead and lucky to be given one more day of life.

PHANTOMS, GHOSTS, AND ALIENS, OH MY!

Mom

Jake began describing his dream to me in the car on our way to his appointment with the psychiatrist. I encouraged him to tell her about it. The moment he said, "lucid dream," she leaned forward a bit and asked him to describe it. He said it felt like he was fully awake in the dream and couldn't escape. Couldn't come out of it.

She asked if he'd noticed any shadowy figures in the dream. He nodded his affirmation. She explained that although there are theories regarding lucid dreams, nothing has been locked in scientifically. There have been studies, of course, and many describe the shadowy figures as phantoms, ghosts, aliens, or just an evil presence. They are none of the above, rather the shadows are all you. She suggested to Jake that he should remember that in such a dream, one's brain wakes up before their body. These dreams happen either upon just falling asleep or in the morning before waking up. She told him to think of it as a gift and to know that he's safe and the figures could just be the edges of his consciousness . . . the edges of waking. He may even be able to enjoy the moment, knowing there's no danger.

I was fascinated by this simple phenomenon and by how complex our brains are. I am still a believer in life being the great equalizer. The pendulum swings back and forth, and there are compensations if you look for them. And believe me . . . I'm looking.

BRAIN WAVES AND VAGUE MEMORIES
Jake

I can't help but wonder about a test I had thirteen or so years ago that read my brain waves. It was called DESA (digital electroencephalogram spectral analyses), and this was its description on the website: "DESA is the recording of electrical patterns at the surface of the scalp, which primarily reflect electrical activity or brainwaves." I was told that I had more sleep waves during the day and more conscious waves at night. What the hell does this even mean for me?

DESA AND THE BLUE GLASSES
Mom

My heart aches as I read Jake's fragile DESA memory. No, it was not a delusion, but another PhD doc that I took Jake to see directly following the release from his first rehab. He had overdosed in sober living, as the psychiatrist they assigned him had given him a strong stimulant medication, then failed to report it to the house manager for safe keeping. Jake had it in his possession.

At any rate, this new educational PhD came with a high recommendation. I brought my frazzled, shell-shocked boy to him and wept openly when he said, "Hang on, Jake. The cavalry is coming."

The following months were full of new medications, odd testing, and peculiar remedies. The DESA, we were told was a brain mapping technology in the form of a brain scan. They put some kind of rubbery skull cap on his head and ran electrodes from there to a machine which displayed colorized images of his brain. I regret letting myself be talked into this, but I was very frightened, and there just wasn't enough information anywhere at this point. A few weeks later, Jake was prescribed a pair of tinted blue glasses to wear for reading, movies, and pretty much everything else. They told us the blue would block out certain colors and make him calmer, less anxious. The glasses had a special name and were expensive. Of course. My bet is that a less costly pair of sunglasses would have done the trick, like the ones he's wearing today from CVS. Plain old light sensitivity.

And so, these weeks and months were filled with experimental tricks and elevated medication that he was taken off when we later went to UCLA for help. The dosage was ridiculously high, and our next doctor had to titrate him down before discontinuing.

The takeaway from all this is that you must never be afraid to say, "Slow down. Explain this to me in a way I can understand," or just plain, "NO." Always use your gut and when something doesn't seem right . . . it isn't right.

Note: *We were told he had Irlen syndrome. Neither the WHO (World Health Organization) nor the DSM-5 (American Psychiatric Assoc) list Irlen's syndrome (or any variant of it) as a recognized disorder.*

STREAM OF CONSCIOUSNESS WHAT IS MY PURPOSE?

Jake

Calm smoking session. Living a dream, my dream of writing with purpose. Why did I live? Why did I dream a dream? If I dream, then why do I dream without purpose? Come on. Dive in. The water is fine. Nude swimming is as close to Nirvana as I can get. Floating penis in mineral rich water. Lots of cream, as thick as it can get. Am I dying? Is my brain slowly fading away? Is my blood pressure so low that I'm not getting enough oxygen to my brain? It seems more important that I write like this rather than trying to make sense. I'm almost positive that the people in the office building where I write are watching what I write. I'm trying to adjust to my Wise-Mind and repeat to myself what the logic of the situation is. Could it be possible that more than one person is hacking into my computer and that the entire place is reading what I write? Not possible. I mean anything is possible, but that it is happening just to me is very unlikely. My therapist would say,

"Why you? Why are you so important?" I can't explain why I would be so important, just that I have a criminal past and that people must keep an eye on me. I believe I have to be totally transparent, and what I'm doing at all times must be monitored by everyone collectively.

Note: *Stream of consciousness writing was for the days Jake was unable to focus because of too many thoughts in his head. He wrote thought to thought without editing or judgement.*

WHAT IS YOUR PURPOSE?
Mom

The truth and Wise-Mind* of it all, my darling son, is that I see how passionately you work at your film, painting, writing, reading, therapy, socializing, and staying on your medication, and with all of this dedication, you will still have these days . . . these moments that will kick your ass and send you back to these familiar obsessive thoughts that cling tight to you.

Thoughts. Random thoughts. You're being watched by a world of people who know all about you. You're a bad person with dark secrets and a criminal life. Your life is coming to an end. The food you eat is being poisoned. None of these are true, Jake. But, this schizophrenia, this illness is on a loop in your brain telling you otherwise. You might shake it off today, but it will be back tomorrow . . . or the next day.

Repeating aloud these paralyzing and false thoughts will bring new truth and set you free. Bring them into the light and they will vanish. Each time, that will be your weapon.

You are so strong, and I will always fight alongside you to bring out the warrior in you. It's in there along with all your creative brilliance. Your purpose, you ask? That's a tough question for anyone. Taking what we are given in life and then to learn and grow is the same for all of us. I believe your purpose is the greater gift.

Wise-Mind is the meeting place in your brain between emotion and solid fact.

CABARET

Jake

I'm writing on my laptop with the sound of rain emanating from an echo dot. My week has been busy. I went to a cabaret show in West Hollywood where my sister Molly and her husband were performing along with fifteen or so other singers. They were songs from James Bond movies. My mom and I arrived around 7:00 p.m. to a charmingly lit restaurant and sat directly in front of the old wood stage. I glanced around me.

My stomach rumbled. I was starving and knew that if I were to eat, I'd have to let go of the paranoia about my food being poisoned. There was a celebrity in the room, the T-1000 from *Terminator 2*, Robert Patrick. Was this a wink-wink moment from the government? Was I to be terminated by the food here? Probably not, I tried to reassure myself.

Just then, a cute blonde waitress approached our table, and I ordered a Coke. I knew I wouldn't want to drink it, but I ordered it anyway. We also ordered appetizers.

The show began and a man in a James Bond tuxedo took the mic. He introduced the first of the singers. I wasn't panicked so far but I expected to be. I was convinced I was going to drop dead in the middle of the show and could honestly feel my heart slowing inside my chest.

Next up was a girl singing the theme from the Bond film *Octopussy*. She was a big breasted, classically beautiful girl. She joked about the title of the song and that in fact, she had eight vaginas. I couldn't help thinking, "If you aren't going to get this woman into bed, then you don't deserve to live."

As she finished her song, I had a small heart flutter that made me gasp for air. Was I going to bite the dust? Not a time for contemplation, so I leaned over to my mom. "I'm going to the bathroom." I got up from my seat and walked past the audience with my head down. In the back of the restaurant was a short hallway with the bathroom at the end. I saw a few of the night's singers hanging out there, including the funny eight-vaginaed girl. I desperately needed a distraction, so I sidled up to her. "Hey, you were great up there."

"Oh, thank you," she smiled sweetly.

"So, do you guys get to choose the songs you sing?"

The girl made a gesture with her hands like handing out paper. "No, they just give it to us and say, go."

"Oh," was all I could say, then turned and walked away; I headed back to the audience. My head was swirling as I put one foot in front of the other. I could've asked for her number or had a longer conversation. I don't know why that happens to me.

Next on stage was my sister's friend Tristan. I had always found him very attractive but couldn't tell if I was truly attracted or just found him handsome on a surface level. It was like reading comprehension in school. It wasn't one of my strengths, and when it came to people, it appeared to be the same.

He began to sing. The song was "Golden Eye," originally sung by Tina Turner, which was one of my all-time favorites. Coincidence? I got chills hearing his rendition. He finished the song and simply said, "Bye," then left the stage. I got up from the table and walked to the other room where he stood leaning over the bar.

"That was awesome," I said, then suddenly I wanted to ask him about my own sexuality and maybe what it was like for him to be gay . . . if he even was. All I could muster was, "Yeah, um . . . you were awesome," then quickly left.

Overall, it was a good night. I was as brave as I could be in a room full of people. I followed my instincts, ignored a lot of paranoid thoughts, and made some stuff happen. So, I suppose my quest continues. Who am I? I don't know how many more opportunities I'm going to have though, to ask out another Octopussy.

HOMEWORK EXERCISE

These are notes from Jake's cognitive behavioral therapist regarding those rough days when you know there will be a social situation that could trigger you:

1. Take your meds early if you can. For me, it was all about my antipsychotic (Clozapine in my case). Just 50 mg before I went out that night would really calm my thoughts.

2. Identify the bad thought and do a reality check.

    a. Remind yourself that thoughts are just thoughts.

    b. Just because you think something, it does not mean it will happen.

    c. And most important is to remind yourself, "I've had this thought many times and it's never happened." You'll be surprised with this one, because those thoughts are on a loop in your head . . . repeating and repeating. They are not real.

DEADLY ORANGE JUICE
Jake

This morning started off as harmless as could be. I woke up, walked to the kitchen, and got some cereal. I saw that the orange juice was out of the fridge and already on the counter. This gave me pause. Was somebody tampering with the orange juice. I had mostly gotten over my paranoia of OJ, but still it lingered, like a bad smell. I grabbed a glass without thinking and poured the remaining liquid into it, then sat and drank it all.

A morning cigarette and Diet Coke is part of my waking up ritual, so I immediately sat on the bench outside my room and lit up. I'd finished about half of the cig when my dad exited the house and looked at me.

"Hey, how's it going today?" he asked easily.

"Good, Dad. Thanks."

I watched him come toward me, then sit on the bench beside me. He had never done this before. "See that tree?"

he asked, "... the bottlebrush. It lost another branch last night. I don't think it's going to make it."

I leaned a bit to the right. "That one back there?"

"Yeah."

Suddenly, I felt myself drifting out of my body. My dad sitting with me, talking about dying trees. I flashed back to the orange juice. Did he find the glass I used to drink it? Did he know I had taken the bait and drunk the poisonous juice? Perhaps he was feeling sorry for me and didn't want me to be alone as I died? I could have stayed with my father and rode out the paranoid wave, but I just couldn't do it. Couldn't take the chance.

"I'll be back in a second," I said, lying.

I went back into my room and lay down on the couch counting each breath. I just couldn't be on that bench with my dad in that moment. It was too scary for me. I felt bad about leaving him like that. I waited and finally heard him get up and go back into the house. I stayed on my couch for an hour or so, and by the time I got up, my shallow breathing had calmed. I was ready for the rest of my day. I'm not sure if I'll ever get rid of my poisoned orange juice fear, but my Wise-Mind tells me that every time I've ever had a drink of it, I've ended up on the other side, living and breathing into another day. I'll try to hang on to that thought for the next time.

ORANGE JUICE AND DAD
Mom

Our kitchen, like most family kitchens, is the heart of our family. Lots of activity, food, and talk. I glanced out the glass door that led to our back patio and saw Jake and his dad sitting on the bench in front of his room. It made me smile. After a few minutes, John came into the house and said they'd had a nice talk. Pleasant and easy. He seemed very pleased.

Jake and his dad have a loving relationship. They don't often sit together and talk feelings. In fact, it's rare. Fairly typical father–son stuff. They watch sports together on occasion and go to action movies that I have no interest in. I love it when they go to Disney Concert Hall to share their love of music or to a play that has sparked Jake's interest. I don't believe there's a great deal of conversation between them during these events, but there is love and there is safety.

I'm no longer surprised by these random moments of irrational fear, like thoughts of being poisoned that plague

Jake. They don't hurt us because they are not about us. They are the illness speaking. Only the symptoms.

What I just read in Jake's words makes me instantly brighten. It is the first time he has written both the fear and resolved it for himself . . . and in less than two pages. After three years of cognitive behavioral therapy, the puzzle pieces are coming together, and I am celebrating his victory.

LOVING KINDNESS MEDITATION

From Jake's cognitive behavior therapist, Jacquelyn. We thank her for this one.

1. Breathe in and out **slowly**.

2. Exhaling and inhaling slowly.

3. Do "Willing Hands." This is simply putting your hands out in front of you on your lap with palms up. Relax.

4. Close your eyes.

5. Quietly say:

   a. "May I be at peace?"

   b. "May I be calm?"

   c. May I be smart?"

Note: *Keep slowly repeating these steps as long as you want.*

TO LET GO OR NOT TO LET GO

Mom

It always seems that Jake sits us down to discuss going on a trip or getting his own apartment during his very worst moments, like after he's secretly skipped one of his medications for several weeks or after he has had a bad bout of paranoia and decided that a bottle of whisky is far better than the debilitating fear that he feels every single day. His goal is to escape. Escape the crushing weight of a thousand random thoughts that strike simultaneously. It's the damn perfect storm of denial, but it connects with seeking freedom. I get it. I really do.

Saying no to our adult son is painful, so John and I repeatedly question ourselves. You might assume that it would be easier to just let him go and live his life as he chooses. Perhaps you'd surmise that it would be the morally right thing to do; after all, he is an adult. It is his right. But there is also a particular responsibility inherent in having a loved one with this illness. In the beginning, I let go a bit more . . . until I realized he might end up on the street or worse. In the beginning, he wasn't medicated; he was in his mid-twenties, and it was hard to tell what was good or bad for him. I was also very scrambled inside as to when and where it had all gone off the rails.

Was it the night he looked at me, eyes brimming with tears, and asked for help?? Was it the night he didn't come home, and we found that he'd slept in an alley? Was it the day I was folding laundry and he came home to tell us that the neighbor in his apartment building was hacking into his computer and spying on him, then asked if I knew something that he'd done that was bad . . . very bad, and that whether I was keeping it from him. What would you do?

MOVING OUT
Jake

I've been trying to find an apartment to live in. I have a chunk of money I've saved up from disability that can cover a year's rent minus living expenses. It's been hard committing to this since there are tons of people looking at the same places as me. Plus, my mother is convinced that I'm not ready to move into a place of my own. I think she's afraid I'll drink myself into a stupor every day with nothing to do and no work to keep me focused. I need to be on my own.

I have a problem with my credit. It's non-existent, and I haven't had a job in over two years, so I'll need to co-sign with my parents. Does anyone even do that anymore? At my age?

There's a property in Encino that seems legit and available. I know I'd love the first few weeks living there. I don't know, maybe I'd get bored. There might be a way I can get my old job back or find video editing work online. I'm certain if I find work, I'll be okay again. I belong to an editing subscription site and pay a monthly fee. I'll finally be able to use it on a professional level.

It's a challenge to navigate the waters of my life when my mom controls everything. I love her more than anything, but sometimes she won't let me make my own mistakes. For example, drinking. She will not allow me to drink while living in her home, which in the long run is understandable, but to be honest, I feel I can control it. I can just see her reacting to this paragraph . . . see the disappointment on her face. "How can you say that?" she might say. "You have absolutely no control over your drinking."

I've gotten to the point where I've been okay without drinking, which makes me wonder, *If I can handle being sober, then can't I handle being loaded?*

Okay, probably not. Anyway, staying sober raises questions that I would've never considered while being loaded. So, I guess I'm still up in the air about sobriety. It's the only thing that quiets my brain.

Freedom in my space has been an issue with my mom for the past five years or so. For instance, in the morning when she wakes me up, she immediately starts cleaning up my room and organizing things—which makes me angry and gets me out of bed. Maybe that's exactly what she wants.

Where are my rights? I had them taken away once at UCLA Resnick Psychiatric, so I know how that feels. Today is difficult for me because I'm tired beyond recognition. I think it's from my new medication. In fact, I know it is.

TO CONTROL OR NOT TO CONTROL
Mom

I know my son feels resentful, if not angry, most of the time at my constant managing of his life. This is a brutally tough issue, especially as he gets older and would in any other circumstance be living freely out in the world . . . good choices or bad, because it is most definitely his life.

I want to let go . . . it is a parent's instinct to let your child fly solo. I will not spend my time or yours defending my actions over these past years, except to say that if given the chance to go back and make different choices when he first began having problems, I would do it the same way. Perhaps, if I did it again though, I would wish for more patience.

I just read those first two paragraphs to Jake and he looked stunned. "Wow," he murmured. I rethought what I'd written. I really do feel that way. He is not on the streets. He is not in jail. Thank God. And he has not been hospitalized once in the past five years. I've thought many times that I need to loosen my grip a bit. Not push so hard at other times. But I see where he is now. How far he's come and how proud that makes him. I hate that it will never be easy for Jake.

It's funny, you know . . . his charge that I control him. There is loads of truth there, of course. I've never been able to accept that he is simply mentally ill with schizophrenia, and therefore, all hope is lost . . . that he can never have relationships or hold a job. He can never accomplish anything. I say, bullshit! Before this illness struck him, he was a wildly creative guy, and we have hundreds of videos from the years before all this; he was a truly beautiful and accomplished boy. I know that's still inside him, and bit by bit, his therapists have found those pieces and brought them back to life. It's hard work and like the movie *Groundhog Day*, with Bill Murray, we find ourselves set back constantly until he finally begins to learn that he might just be able to stay the course. And that makes it all worthwhile.

Jake, you talk a lot about finding an apartment and nothing about what really worries us. What will you do at night when your paranoia comes back? Will you choose the fastest method . . . drinking, to drown out the thoughts, to blot out the world, which will also derail your meds that keep your brain quiet? And ultimately, will you remember to take your medication every day without letting your brain tell you that it's okay to do less or none at all?

I want this for you too. This freedom to live your own life on your own terms. Where are your pros and cons? What is the plan? Do you think you can ignore your brain telling you that you can, in fact, handle drinking? That you can occasionally skip medication? That it's okay to miss your doctor appointments?

Specific plan of action! I know you can do this.

MOVING OUT
(LAST WORD)

Jake

If at night I feel a panic attack coming on preceded by dark and threatening thoughts, I'll take a walk outside, maybe even find someone who is around to talk to. Definitely dive into a creative project, video editing or painting. I don't think drinking will be the first solution. I've been taking all my meds including my new medication, even though you don't believe I have. If I feel paranoid about that, I can call my therapists and see if they're available to talk. What are the pros and cons of having a place to live on my own?

Cons: Being alone. At night. Needing to talk with someone when I need it . . . right now. Paranoia about neighbors. Are they talking about me?

Pros: Being on my own and free to be creative by myself. No one telling me what to do or when to do it. Being able to be social and bring new people home to my own place. Make my own mistakes and set my own course. To cook naked.

SELECTIVE PARANOIA

Jake

"I have schizophrenia. I am not schizophrenia. I am not my mental illness. My illness is a part of me."

—Jonathan Harnisch

I worry about things that years of therapy have taught me are not real or harmful to me, like poisoned food. There are days on end when I can eat only packaged food. I have trouble going back to unfinished drinks because I'm afraid someone has put something in them when I left the room, or my back was turned. By morning, there are six to ten half-empty soda cans left around the house that I will never touch. I can't.

I'm afraid of my heart failing. I fixate on my stomach and chest to see it rise and fall as my heart beats. By the end of the day when my heart slows to a lower rate, it is a completely terrifying time for me. I fear going to sleep because

I know my heart will stop beating entirely. I lose connection with my body.

I fear cameras, computers, and television on my bad days, as they represent my infamy. Everyone knows everything about me.

Cognitive behavioral therapy has taught me to find my logical mind. What is true? What is real? These three areas are not based on logic. I will face them down every day of my life, and I will use my logic to banish them.

While I obsess over these terrors, I all but ignore the fact that I smoke profusely, overeat like crazy, and down Red Bull and sugary drinks all day. All things that are realistically harmful to me—cancer, obesity, and diabetes—why am I not obsessing about those things? It's what my mom calls selective paranoia. A silly paradox that I live with every day.

WHISTLING
Jake

I am thankful and happy that my parents don't whistle to intentionally get on my nerves. Or to scare me. I'm not sure when it began, but for at least three years, people who recognized me . . . from the massage parlor porn . . . from the cameras in my parent's house, have whistled whenever I've walked into a room they occupied. How do I know it's about me? Because people don't whistle in real life. They whistle in movies. They whistle in songs. But random out-of-nowhere whistling is pretty rare, isn't it? I'm still not sure why people whistle in my face. Is it because they hate me and want to annoy me? Is it because they're scared of me and want me to back off?

I recently went to a Starbucks register to pay for my items. The employee looked happy and was enjoying a laugh with another barista. Then he glanced up at me, and out came a one-note whistle blow. It must've lasted at least five seconds. At first, it scared me. What did this whistle mean? He seemed like a nice guy. But was he?

The other time it bothers me is when it's a family member. Recently during a summer dinner, my brother-in-law Michel whistled after a conversation with my sister and me. I remember asking her if anything I'd said was offensive. She said, no, of course not, and that was that. I was afraid that maybe she'd told him about it because a few minutes later, he was back, whistling intensely. That got to me, made me angry . . . scared. Thankfully, it was brief.

I'm trying to remember that it's only a whistle and not a big deal at all. As Bacall said to Bogart, ". . . just put your lips together and blow."

JUST WHISTLE IT AWAY
Mom

Whistling. How could I have missed that trigger? But then I realize, your very admission in writing tells me that you're getting better. Heading in the right direction. Last year, you couldn't even voice your fears or trigger words. That was simply too terrifying. Now, thoughts from the darkest part of your mind are beginning to be shared and brought safely into the light.

One of your great-grandmothers was a big whistler, so yes, people do whistle. She annoyed everyone because she was always out of tune and her whistle was wiggly with a broad vibrato. We'd groan and bury our heads . . . but it brought laughter, not fear.

I might do a long whistle at random now and then as a sign of exasperation or maybe a blast of hyper energy. That last one happens less often for me now, but make no mistake . . . whistling is mostly random. It's hardly an art.

Snow White and the dwarves whistled a plenty. They marched happily to the mines singing "Heigh-Ho" and

76

whistling, while Snow White whistled "a happy tune" as she worked cleaning their cottage. All cheery references.

I know when your ears sometimes hear someone on a street, mall, or lobby whistling, your brain immediately tells you that this is a message meant only for you, and it brings danger. Logic here? It is not for you, or about you. It is not a warning or a hidden message. It is simply a silly moment for that person, like someone sighing, laughing, or talking to themselves . . . about nothing in particular.

Remember what I did when you were little and you woke from a nightmare? Take the fear in your hands. Crush it between your palms . . . then blow the dust into the wind.

THE GIRL AND GLENDALE
Jake

I was more depressed than I realized while dating a girl from my outpatient facility in Glendale. Oh, I enjoyed our time together and mostly felt good being around her; she was beautiful but intensely co-dependent. There were also times I felt she could replace me with anyone. She was holding on to contact with her ex-boyfriend while he texted her something like thirty times a day. I asked her if she would break it off, but she refused. Somewhere inside, she was convinced that I would leave her, and so she needed that backup.

I ignored my alcohol issues back then and would drink heavily with this girl at her apartment. I knew something was wrong with me, and the drinking was probably just an off-shoot. One night we shared a bottle of vodka, and it got out of control. I had never been a loud or belligerent drunk . . . mostly quiet, keeping to myself, like tonight. Silent, no energy, no focus . . . just that heavy cloud surrounding me.

I hid in the bathroom with a sharp kitchen knife and began to cut at my wrists. I wanted to see how far I could go without killing myself. I wasn't sure what she was doing outside the door . . . Was she calling the police?

Suddenly, there were voices. Loud, in my head. *"You fucking loser. You can't keep a relationship going without drinking yourself into a black hole."* With that, I got the blood flowing with one cut; a piece of ragged skin I flayed off my wrist, then grabbed a corner and pulled it the rest of the way. *"What are you doing to yourself? You don't even have the guts to follow through,"* the voice continued to berate me. *"Do it!!! Kill yourself!!!"*

I finally made my way outside the bathroom where I found her crouched along the wall. The sight made me cry. "I don't know what I'm doing . . ."

She lunged at me, grabbed the knife from my hands, and carried it to the kitchen. In a daze, I trailed after her. I can't recall anything clearly, but I do know that it was her idea to cut herself. To cut ourselves together. So much alcohol between us. I'd watched her, knife in hand, try to slice her own wrist; although strangely, in the end, there was only a small scrape on her.

Tremendous confusion that night and of course I had no medication inside me. The booze had driven it all out. She screamed that she had called the police. It was at this point that I knew I had no control, so I grabbed my jacket and left her apartment. I didn't have a car, so I just ran, up the street and around the corner. . I jumped a fence behind her building and landed hard on the backs of my heels. The pain was unbelievable. That was when I dropped down on the sidewalk. I had nothing to prove. Nothing left to say. My mind was spinning. Twenty minutes passed and the faint sound of a siren woke me.

The next thing I knew, I was on my way to Glendale Hospital to be locked up for an undisclosed amount of time. It was a cold dark place, all blues and greens.

It was to be my second time in a facility. No, third, including Alhambra. There were at least two "lifers" in the ward that were beyond help. At least that's the way I remember it. Not much else to recall other than the "girlfriend" showing up and making sure I was okay. At the time, it made me happy, having her there, as if she wasn't afraid of me and that she was there for me no matter what. We talked that day, during visiting hours in the outside area and planned to move in together permanently. Then . . . she brought out engagement rings. An awkward moment to propose to somebody. Bizarre even. We hadn't known each other long. Weeks? A couple of months? But for some reason, it was a huge relief. I felt that if we were together, nothing else could harm us.

A MOTHER'S NIGHTMARE
Mom

That whole week had been a nightmare. The perfect storm of chaos surrounding Jake. He was unmedicated, in an alcohol-dependent cloud, lonely, frustrated, and terrified. This was the summer of 2013. He'd just spent a month at the Betty Ford Center getting sober, although his struggles went well beyond their wheelhouse of twelve-step structure. They were compassionate and educated in their approach as well as fully aware that he needed a place that functioned as a dual diagnosis facility. What they did offer was an on-site psychiatrist who was the first doctor to diagnose Jake with schizophrenia. He claimed to be "99 percent certain."

Jake's account of the night in Glendale from his point of view is a powerful memory, and I absolutely cringe as I read it. Of course, I wasn't there in that apartment, so knowing the details of what was going on in his head that night makes my heart beat faster. My own memory really begins with a phone call from the girl at 2:00 a.m. "I've locked myself in the bathroom," she began, whispering. "There's blood every-where." Talk about shock. Her words nauseated me.

"Where is Jake??? What happened?" She was both dra-matic and maddeningly vague. I had never trusted her. Too much had happened. This girl had parked in front of our home just a week ago, hysterical and sobbing as she told our son that if he broke up with her, she would kill herself. We called the police and by the time they walked to the window of her car, she had miraculously changed to a dry-eyed intelligent businesswoman capable of producing proof of employment and stability. She flashed me a look and smiled as my husband and I stood behind the officers. I was terrified of the power this girl held over Jake when he was so vulnerable. Within a few weeks of meeting him in the outpatient rehab, she'd given him a ring to wear, told him she wanted to have his babies, then weeks after that, emailed him a bill for gifts she'd given him while they dated. She crushed him. She texted me threats and attempted to blackmail all of us.

Still parked with Jake in front of our house, she soon con-vinced him to go back home with her, even after I tried to reason that he needed to be closer to his doctor for a few weeks and get back on his medication. The officer pulled me aside. He spoke with kindness and sympathy. His hands were tied. Jake was an adult. We had to watch him drive off with her, and now here was the call in the middle of the night.

We got in our car and drove silently and quickly to her address downtown. As we approached the block she lived in, there were flashing red lights of police cars, a firetruck, and paramedics on the far corner. Maybe it was 3:00 a.m. by then. Jake's dad had trouble finding a place to park, so he stopped for a moment . . . I jumped out and bolted at a dead run toward the lights. It seemed endless, like in a nightmare where you run and run and run and it keeps getting farther away. Jake had never gotten into trouble in his life, and all my mother's instincts were on fire. Death by cop? What was happening?

I got to the corner and saw him with the officer. Jake's hands were behind his back as they stood by the hood of the police car. I quickly stepped off the curb, but the cop warned me off. "Stay where you are."

My heart was pounding in my ears. Jake's dad appeared behind me and took my shoulders, then gently held my hand. The girl walked up to us and whispered her reminder that Jake had tried to get her to cut her wrists, so maybe she might just tell the cop. She hadn't decided. Her breath wreaked of alcohol. Jake told us later that she'd made a pact with him to do it together but backed out.

We looked over at Jake. He was clearly loaded, but worse, he was psychotic. I knew the look. It's that step beyond drunk. Frail and wild-eyed. He was also angry that she had called the police. He was instructed to sit on the curb while both officers reassured us that he had done nothing illegal, and they would not press charges. However, they immediately put him on a psych hold and the EMTs were there to take him to the hospital. His wrists were dripping blood beneath the loose bandages, but they assured me it didn't appear life threatening. He was limping badly, and we would find that he'd gotten a hairline fracture on his heel when he jumped over her fence. He also needed stitches in his wrist where he'd nicked an artery in his cutting. We waited with him for nine hours to get a bed because there was confusion regarding his insurance. Big surprise.

This hospital ER was stunning. Clean, white, and well-run. It looked like it had been recently remodeled. I was grateful he was here. They finally figured out his insurance, and John and I walked beside his wheelchair as they took him up to the psych floor. If you have ever seen *The Wizard of Oz*, then you'll remember the moment when Dorothy steps out of her house after the cyclone. Her world goes from black and white to brilliant color. Well, reverse that. We left the brilliantly gleaming ER and walked down the first hallway past new rooms and smiling nurses. There was a short elevator ride, and we got off on a floor that was older. Drab even. My gut clutched as we approached the doors at the end of the long hall. Inside was a room straight out of the 1950s. Dingy linoleum floors, old cabinets, gray metal folding chairs, and a much-used table like you'd see in an old cafeteria. There was nothing on the gray walls. Not one thing. My throat clutched. This is where I'm to leave my despondent child? We weren't even allowed to walk him to his shared room. It took everything in me not to scream. We promised him we would be back during visiting hours in the morning.

This is mental illness. This is how they are treated. Wouldn't you think that a bright room, filled with light and color on the walls might help a little? A minor thought at such a moment, but astounding in its simplicity. How much would a few posters cost? Surely, we have slipped back in time when having a brain disease is a life sentence of shame and misery with no rights and most likely confinement to a lunatic asylum.

But no, this moment was in 2013. We must fight harder and longer for our loved ones. It's difficult for me to find the time or strength to fight in Congress for better laws, so, for now . . . I write. We reach out to you so that you know someone else has walked this path. I see Jake today and he is seated at his desk writing this book inside our well-lit office here in Studio City and I know there is hope. He fights it all day, every day. At least here, he can feel safe. Here he can express himself and focus on helping someone like himself. Never give up.

THE GIRL AND GLENDALE
A LAST THOUGHT
Jake

Reliving the events of that night is brutal, not only because I have deep regrets but because my memory sucks. Years of medication has dimmed all perceptions. At the time, I thought I had a friend in her, but really, all that remains is shame, which sadly blankets everything.

DAYS OF THUNDER
Mom

I try not to anticipate or assume anymore when it comes to each day, because schizophrenia dictates its own erratic course. One time, my sister Marilyn looked at me in the middle of one of my angst-driven days and suggested I try for "acceptance" a little more often. Life makes more sense this way in general, but for as long as I can remember, hope has been my guiding light and that pushes me well beyond the confines of acceptance.

The early years of the illness taught us that three good days was often followed by a splattering of white-knuckled chaos. It's still that way, but the difference now is that Jake has indeed improved over all. But like how it is with a smoker or alcoholic who is only one cigarette or one glass of booze away from disaster, so it is with schizophrenia. One trigger word, one unexpected thought that consumes him, one new medication that tips the scales, and we are back to square one. Or almost. He seems to hang on by his fingernails, and that is the miracle. I am not so resilient and seem to have gathered more impatience and a degree of desperation along the way.

As I write this in my own tempered chaos, I realize I will always choose hope and Jake will always have me at his coattails, pushing him, perhaps a bit harder than I should. Therein lies the hope.

SHAME

Jake

Do you feel shame? Aren't you going to put away the potato chips? I get up from my seat and grab the bag, wondering if my thoughts come from some kind of real place. Is shame something I must create out of necessity? Do I create it for the people around me so they will feel more comfortable? Or do I do it because it's so ingrained in my personality, in my brain?

One time an ex-girlfriend asked me, "How do you organize the thoughts in your head?" It was as though she thought I was a librarian telling her to go to *aisle G7* for information. I'll never be certain of my personality, having only lived (and will ever live) inside one head.

Another girl I went on a date with told me bluntly, ". . . it's as if you're not a real person." What did that even mean? I wasn't ready to respond to something so random back then. Only now am I ready to figure out what she meant. I was told by another friend that she thought I had a borderline personality disorder. I should mention that she had just started taking psychology at the local Valley College. She wrote a school paper on me, like I was a pet project.

Some psychologist told me she thought I had mild Asperger's. Then finally came the big one; I was told that I had schizophrenia, during my rehab stint at The Betty Ford Clinic. That was a shocker.

After all of that, how am I supposed to trust that there is a true diagnosis when it's all over the place? I guess you can chalk it up to the spectrum disorder. It's the latest popular mental disorder term . . . or maybe it's been around for a while and finally the word just caught on. Damn the spectrum. Damn it all to hell.

My mom just handed me a term she had read, which is a symptom of schizophrenia. Anosognosia, which is a lack of insight into your own illness. I'd love to commit to one diagnosis . . . fewer symptoms. I don't think that's too much to ask. Go ahead and label my behaviors and I'll see if I can change them.

OPPOSITE ACTION

Suggestions from Jake's cognitive behavioral therapist for times when your emotions don't fit the facts.

Every emotion has an **action** urge. Change the emotion by acting the **opposite**.

Fear urge: to run away   **Opposite:** approach

Anger urge: to attack   **Opposite:** gently avoid/be kind

Sadness urge: withdraw/isolate   **Opposite:** get active

Shame urge: hide/avoid   **Opposite:** tell a secret to someone who will accept

MY FIRST HOSPITALIZATION
Jake

I sat huddled in the back seat of my dad's 1981 Jeep Grand Wagoneer in the parking lot of the UCLA Neuropsychiatric Hospital. It was dark outside, and I could hear my parents whispering in the front seat.

The building was dimly lit. We were at a distance of a hundred feet, and I could see twenty or so people inside, sitting, pacing, talking . . . waiting to get in to see someone. The psych business was booming. I was terrified of walking in and strongly considered bolting from the car and running for the hills. Instead, I just said, "I don't want to go."

I had done a full 180 since leaving the house and suddenly, that seemed like it might have been the better option. Safe. Home. We three sat in silence. Finally, my mom spoke up and somehow convinced me to go inside to . . . "just take a look."

From the moment I walked through the doors of the UCLA ER, I have little memory of the events that followed. I've been told of the long wait, **the 5150**,* and ultimately the journey by ambulance to another hospital. I suppose it should concern me that there are blank spaces in my brain. These were traumatic times, but if I'm being truthful, it doesn't really bother me because I was so messed up in my head during those days. Wouldn't you want to forget?

*5150 Hold: *This allows an officer or mental health professional to involuntarily commit an individual for seventy-two hours for evaluation if they are a danger to themselves or others.*

SNAKE PIT
Mom

Jake was on a gurney in the hallway because the ER was packed that night. His dad and I took turns sleeping in a nearby chair while the other stayed close to Jake. We spent the next sixteen hours waiting for a bed to open up in the psychiatric ward. A particularly unfeeling nurse demanded blood from our "psychotic" son, and when he fearfully declined, she pointed at a burly security guard and said she would summon him to hold Jake down while she put the needle in him.

Jake quickly rose from the bed and clutched his jacket into a ball in front of him. He moved haltingly toward the exit doors, a cornered animal—the story was all in his eyes. I literally backed that nurse across the room, telling her if she EVER spoke to my boy or any other mentally ill patient in that way again, she would be answering to me.

The past three to four hours in the ER were spent in a small back room with security guards at the door. They'd called a 51'50, which allowed them to keep him there against his will for up to seventy-two hours for psychiatric evaluation. This is something he needed for his own safety. I knew that, so it was somewhat of a relief. If not for that hold, Jake could've left the building on his own. He wasn't eating or sleeping and was convinced that he was about to die either by poison or his heart stopping. There was always the fear of a gunshot wound to his head as he slept.

The month preceding this, he had set his alarm for every fifteen to thirty minutes all night long. By doing this, he could never reach a deep sleep where he felt he would surely die. He was barely eating and was rail thin. Anything I prepared, Jake felt might be tainted. This went on for more than six weeks until the night I knew we had to get him into a hospital as soon as we could. The psychiatrist he'd seen on occasion through his twenties had advised us that it was time to take him in for evaluation and to go directly to the ER.

As dawn approached, two psychiatrists finally appeared to speak with Jake. He told them that he was being poisoned and that he knew his heart would stop at any moment. They asked him if he was angry at us for putting him in there and had he thought of hurting us. I still remember, he looked all of twelve years old, flushed, and wide-eyed with surprise. "I would never hurt my family," he whispered back. My heart swelled and my throat ached. I did not know what was wrong that day, or that he would one day be told that he had schizophrenia, but I will break the urban legend here that says schizophrenia's defining symptom is violence. This is false. In fact, it remains a low risk, somewhere around 6 percent.

At the end of sixteen hours, we were informed that there were still no beds available at UCLA and that Jake would be taken by ambulance to another psychiatric hospital forty-five miles away. We were panicked. Where were they taking him? Would he be cared for as thoroughly without being here at this mainstream hospital? I got in the ambulance beside his gurney. His dad followed in the car. By now, Jake was groggy from the medication they'd given him. When we arrived, I was taken to a waiting area.

The next three days were a nightmare. I couldn't help but recall a 1948 film starring Olivia de Havilland, called *Snake Pit*—a story of a woman who finds herself in an insane asylum and cannot remember how she got there. In the film, we learn she has schizophrenia, but in those days, it was all about electroshock and straitjackets. She was finally tossed into a large, padded cell, the snake pit, with like patients, and abandoned there without hope. This image haunted me.

We sat there, waiting to see our son on that first night. Finally, he was brought down the hall to speak to us, and we all sat in a tiny room, the size of a broom closet. It had no windows, nothing on its drab walls, and only two sticky metal folding chairs inside. The person who brought him, vanished, leaving the three of us alone in the small room. Jake looked terrible: hair wild and eyes darting about him trying to make sense of where he was; the dissolving Zyprexa tablet that he was given at UCLA was wearing off. I was suddenly uncertain of what the hell we were doing there. We wanted to take him home. But it was too late for that. He was held there by law, and we dealt with it as best we could.

It seemed the people brought in on gurneys that were pushed past us were mostly people off the streets. This couldn't be the right place for our son, among those weathered faces that spoke in incoherent murmurs. Were they someone else's lost child from long ago? By now, Jake was even worse than yesterday when we'd first arrived at UCLA. I was sick to my stomach. He looked so frightened and lost. Why wasn't there some place to take him that felt safe? A place that knew what they were doing and had compassion of any form. They were suddenly a part of the problem, and we were all trapped.

I found an old email that I'll share with you. I sent it to Jake's UCLA psychiatrist, Dr. DeAntonio after he'd spent two days there.

"Jake's admitted at Alhambra. Watching them try multiple drugs with no more than 24 hours in between to see if they work . . . then seeing him tonight completely miserable, desperate to escape his mental condition, certain that this place is not for him and saying they're trying to kill him, etc. etc. He told me his brain is shutting down and he wished I could understand how it feels . . . like torture waiting for 'it' to happen. He lingered by the exit door saying goodbye to me tonight . . . begging to go home and when it opened, he walked out as I stood there. Didn't run. Just that 'deer in the headlights' look. The four young psych assistants that ran out to get him seemed like it was more a lark to them than a serious breach of security. I stood there frozen, watching them round him up as they laughed, finally escorting him back inside past me.

"Here is my question given all the information, his condition and possible release tomorrow. If this were your son, would you just have him transferred back to your NPI and damn the cost because that's what I'm thinking. We don't have the money or insurance but will figure it out. I just need

to know if you think this would be the best thing for him. I'm reeling right now from seeing him this way. P.S. Is it right that they use both Cogentin and Haldol then bounce to Risperdal the next?"

With Jake back inside, out of my reach, I walked to my car and cried. This is what happens when you have a mental illness. There is no one who is treated with less dignity than the mentally ill. Not in this place anyway.

After many calls and three days there, Jake had dodged or refused all medication, begged to go home, then with no notification to the family, they released him. I would not have known except for the kind young nurse who called me, whispering into the phone that Jake had been put in a cab with a voucher and taken to an address he'd given them. She said she'd get in trouble for telling us. The address Jake had was his last apartment, and we'd already moved his furniture out, so there was no place for him to go. Our son-in-law Michel called the taxi company, and they tracked the cab's destination. Jake's sister Becky met him and brought him home. UCLA would be our next stop.

STREAM OF CONSCIOUSNESS
*FLUID WRITING AS EACH THOUGHT OCCURS. NO EDITS.
SUBCONSCIOUS ELOQUENCE

Jake

Stream of haunchsciousness. Get positioned. Ready for the old one-two. Ready for the fantastical ass reaming. Don't try to rhyme, don't even try to think. Just pretend you're a free-style rapper. Feeling the flow. Destroying all in your wake. All free falling on the edges of your topcoat. Magician. What is the female version? Magaicain? Magiciaii? Where did it all go wrong? Twenty-three? Twenty-five? Thirty-one? I'm pretty sure it was twenty-five. I've gone back to that moment, the moment hundreds of times. And it wasn't the hit and run. It was much worse than that. Something you don't want to end up in prison for. Elegy. Lament for the dead. A real honest-to-goodness poem. Something Jim Morrison would've recited to the love of his life on a balcony in Venice Beach. But not this. No, thank you. Never this. Is insecurity attractive in a poem? It depends on the person reading I suppose. I suppose, you suppose. What the hell is going on? I feed you, my subconsciousness. Feed it in no particular order. Have to refocus on the subject. Subject being eloquence, and sometimes mental health. Maybe eloquence is more important to me than anything. Why? It seems like an important thing to bring up. It's my theory that if I just took it down 50 percent of the time, took down my eloquence and linguistics energy, I'd be 100 percent happier.

ON THE LEDGE

Jake

Last night was an unexpected horror. Early in the evening, I anticipated all of it . . . a panic attack . . . paranoia. I felt it coming so I went over the script I'd worked on with my therapist. It's a written paragraph we'd put together of my biggest fears. They were always the same.

The idea is that you read the script so many times that you become numb, desensitized to the scary words and thoughts. I went over it a dozen times, which I learned wasn't enough for me.

So, last night, I sat in the living room with my parents watching television, and for whatever reason, the screen went black. There was silence, then my mom just said, "Boom." This seems like such a trivial thing now but at that particular moment, it meant I was going to be shot in the head . . . in my sleep . . . and my mother couldn't help but allude to it. I latched onto the emotion of the moment and was instantly terrified. Convinced that everyone, including our neighbors . . . and my dad knew about all of it. Of course, it happened that the neighbors were having a party just then, with loud music, and I could hear their voices carrying over the fence. I was certain that they were watching a live feed of my life on television or the Internet. It seemed that whenever I stepped outside the kitchen door to have a cigarette, there was a burst of laughter; then more laughter coupled by a "Shhh." This had to be a concerned person, worried for my well-being, so he tried to quiet the one who was making a joke about my impending death. There was a sudden shift inside me. I went from cold stillness to utter certainty that this was going to happen tonight.

I sat beside my mom and tried to make sense of it. I told her about the text message I'd just sent to my sister. I wanted Molly to see a video I'd been working on for her, so I had simply typed, "I sent the link!"

All at once, I wasn't sure what the meaning of my own "sent" message was. It seemed to have a double meaning . . . nefarious. My mom gently reminded me that the message was from my own brain and that it was not logical to think someone could take my own thoughts and change the meaning. Logic.

At this point, I was out of my gourd. I couldn't react to anything she was saying. Just responding with a head nod or a blink . . . a hand to my face. My mind was scrambled and I was grasping at slippery rungs on a ladder.

My mother has a great deal of experience talking me off the ledge of paranoia and always reminds me to think of the image of a person leaning into their fear. ". . . as if it's a wall of wind," she'd say. People in movies who look up at the sky and scream, "What do you want from me?!" Daring the nightmare to finish the job. She reminds me I've used this device in my own movies when Molly or my best friend were in danger and would yell at the top of their lungs. She reminds me that I have that defense mechanism inside me and just need to remember that it's there. Lean into my fear. Today, that is the hope I cling to.

SEEKING YODA
Mom

I wish I could tell you there's an easy answer for what you're going through, a checklist of carefully defined points that apply precisely to you, because mental illness is complicated, make no mistake of that. This world is still decades behind figuring it all out. You will become the expert on your loved one's well-being. There are no definite answers, and oh, so many opinions. There are multitudes of books on mental illness as well as the offshoots from every corner of the spectrum. I think what I hoped to find was a handbook in **large bold print** that didn't give me multiple options for helping my son, rather a book that gave me THE exact roadmap out of this insanity. I longed to be told with great assurance by someone brilliant and titled, what the journey would be from beginning to end. And most important was my need to know that there was a light at the end of this tunnel . . . one that tells me that my boy will get well and be able to follow his dreams again.

It literally took me years to make peace with this thing called schizophrenia. Right from the start, I was a fighter, but

I don't believe I knew what the battle was. Jake was diagnosed with so many things over the first few years by this doctor and that, so you must be ready. Diagnoses began for Jake with GA (generalized anxiety), followed by low level depression, attention deficit disorder, obsessive compulsive disorder, alcoholism, psychosis, Asperger's syndrome, major depression with psychosis, and ultimately schizophrenia. So, you see why we were a bit gun-shy about that final label. Not my child. They had to be wrong. I found it hardest to accept on the good days when Jake was more present than usual, more of the person I knew in childhood.

Like any other problem in life, we have learned to take it one day at a time. So very Alcoholics Anonymous of me. The truth is in the simplicity. You'll hear me use that phrase often.

So, what is my advice? Read all you can about the illness. Study the medications so that you are a part of the decision-making team. I know that Jake is lightweight with meds, and they hit him hard, so doses need to be low and titrated up slowly. We learned he cannot handle stimulants such as Adderall or Concerta. These make his head feel clearer, so he immediately takes more. Anything addictive like this is bad for him. Every time we went to a new doctor, I had to argue that point again and again. They'd look at me as a controlling parent. I can't begin to count the number of times I was hit with "enabler" or "too involved" during his rehab stints. Accept that banner without hesitation because you are the only thing standing between your child and the system, which is poorly regulated, underrepresented, and universally misunderstood.

We were all shocked seeing Jack Nicholson in *One Flew Over the Cuckoo's Nest*, which culminated with his character receiving a lobotomy. The novel was published in 1962, and the movie came out in 1975. More than forty-five years later, we are still whispering about mental illness. A cure for schizophrenia has often been promised within five or ten years, but by the end of that time, nothing has really changed as there is never enough funding for research, even though 1.5 million will be diagnosed with schizophrenia this year, worldwide.

Read about deinstitutionalization in the 1970s. Many of the people released from those "insane asylums" ended up on the streets, unmedicated and homeless. To this day, we have not solved that problem; our streets in Los Angeles are loaded with the homeless, and our jails are 44 percent mentally ill. The NAMI support groups I occasionally attend are filled with parents of these lost souls in our jails. They come without direction or hope, and their eyes are as lost as their children. As a group, we feel more powerful because we share our experiences and knowledge.

In the end, you will not come upon your helper, your Yoda, on a list of doctors or hospitals. It will take time and patience and an eye for the one who "gets it," then you will know this is your person. Until it isn't. The battle will continue. Build your team. One at a time. A psychiatrist. Then hopefully a great cognitive behavioral therapist. There are bad ones, so watch out. We've fallen into that pit. I found our magical therapist ten years ago, and we instantly knew to hang on because Jake could talk to her at those times when he was certain that his heart won't keep him alive until the end of the day. He is safely at home with us each night and we support him in his search for relief from his symptoms. There is a point where I feel I actually am that Yoda, the wise one, who keeps him on a path that will one day lead to his mental freedom. I pray that is true.

DISTRACTION IS THE KEY
Mom

The first time I became aware of using distraction to help Jake was the day he was released from Alhambra. I drove him back to Resnick Neuropsychiatric Hospital at UCLA. He was fragile, as was I, considering the debacle of the past few days.

Dr. DeAntonio was Jake's psychiatrist at UCLA. He had been seeing Jake occasionally over the past couple of years for depression. That day, he told me to bypass the ER and take him straight up to fourth floor psych, as they'd be expecting us. As we pulled into the big circular driveway out front, I saw there was a valet service. Thank God. I remember getting out of the car first. The entire trip over the hill from the San Fernando Valley, Jake had been frightened and agitated about where I was taking him. Understandably, he didn't want to go anywhere, and his eyes began darting right and left for an escape. I braced myself for complete resistance.

As I stood outside the car, he remained rooted to the passenger seat inside, clearly freaking out. This felt impossible.

My own panic was rising. What if I couldn't get him inside? There was no way I would take him home in this state. I feared for his safety, and I didn't want anyone to physically force him to go in. If I left him for a minute to go find help, he'd disappear in a red-hot second.

Then, without another thought, I dropped my keys on the ground, so they landed just underneath my side of the car. "Shit, I dropped my keys. Jake, can you see them?" I asked, letting him hear my distress. He slowly got out of the car and began looking around. "I see them," he said; by then, he was walking around to my side. We both crouched and retrieved them. I laughed and just kept talking about how dumb it was that I couldn't seem to hang on to my keys . . . losing them sometimes or misplacing. Soon, we were moving across the big hospital lobby. He was nervous of course, but I kept him thinly engaged. "Do you ever do that?" I asked him, still keeping my eyes on his face to watch for signs. "Wow, this lobby is huge. Do you remember where we're supposed to go?"

I rattled on this way until we reached the fourth floor. I continued to keep his brain busy. Distraction only works with sincerity and calm. I found asking a question automatically engaged his brain, keeping it from negative thoughts, so it was clear I had to make it good. With schizophrenia, each person will deal with a unique set of symptoms and personality traits, so going with your gut is imperative.

I still use distraction when Jake is building to a panic. It's a skill each family will need to help your loved one escape the worst moments in their head. Jake and I talk about it now in hopes that he can learn to be his own distractor. His own man. I admire that he never seems to dwell on what this illness has taken from him, rather how to find peace. There have been days and weeks when I sense he feels defeated and turns to alcohol or skipping meds or both, but in the grand scheme, he seems to be on the road to freedom. It's riddled with holes and detours, but finding that road is half the battle.

Are there times that I doubt myself? Fear that I'm hurting more than helping? Oh, hell yes. Every day. The years have gone by and I'm aware at times that my life has morphed into something I don't recognize, but at the same time, there is an unexplained richness and wisdom one acquires when you experience life on deeper levels. Today, at the moment of this writing, I still believe we are blessed beyond measure. That might sound odd, but there it is.

ESCAPE

Jake

The UCLA psych hospital had three or four narrow compartments, all laid out like the interior of train cars; each compartment was separated by a pneumatic sliding door and held different levels of mental patients. I would be right next door to the worst-off patients in the end car. I wondered how bad it got there. Patients smearing their excrement on walls? The truth of the matter was that most patients there were not as bad as you'd imagine. Just, lost. Lost socially. Lost in their own family. Lost in their heads.

There were six or seven rooms per compartment, each the size of a small hotel room. My name had already been printed out and taped to the door's small glass window. It was spelled out with lower and uppercase letters.

jAkE

I had seen people write to me in emails and Facebook this way. Did this trigger some kind of subconscious response like *The Manchurian Candidate*? The names on other doors were properly printed. James. Katie. Ned. I never asked anyone why, even though it bothered me. Scared me even. But then everything scared me at the time.

After the narrow tour of the premises, I sat on my room's hospital bed with my mom. She seemed almost enthusiastic about the admittance, although I couldn't be sure what she was thinking. She took my hand, and I took a deep breath. One of the nurses walked in the room and handed me a fifty-question psyche packet to fill out. She also gave me a menu of different foods to order for breakfast, lunch, and dinner for the entire week, so I knew I wasn't leaving soon. As I glanced down the list, I was terrified. I didn't want to eat anything that wasn't packaged. I was sure that someone would poison my food if I wasn't making it myself. The only packaged option was kosher, and that was what I would eat my entire stay. There was also a small refrigerator in the central room we all shared. I would eat from that as it was consistently restocked with wrapped tuna and ham sandwiches, yogurt, and ice cream.

There weren't many other patients there and, to my disappointment, only one female. In my rehab experiences in the past, the best friends I made were girls.

This female was almost completely isolated and hardly ever out of her room. When she did appear in the hallway, I felt guilty that I didn't try to talk with her.

There were visible security cameras in my hallway. I counted ten throughout the entire compartment from the monitor I saw at the nurse's station. I did a lot of pacing during my stay there. Back and forth . . . back and forth. From one end of the hallway to the other. I felt like a trapped animal, but it was the only thing to do to get any relief. I eventually discovered a relaxation room at the other end of the hallway. It had one small bed and four walls with a beach mural on it. The isolation helped a bit but mainly made me want to get out of there. To a real beach. To anywhere.

Once a week, there was a small group of doctors who strolled through the ward, stopping at each door to observe the patients. Eventually, they got to my door. There was a group of five. Only one of them talked. "How are you doing, Jake?" he asked. I didn't know what to say. They all seemed cold and procedural.

"How are you doing?" I asked back, then, "How long does the average person stay here?" I wanted to know.

"Well, you'll be staying here until you . . ." the doctor appeared to seize up, his arms in a frozen position, and he gave a small laugh. Was it a laugh? He smiled at his coworkers, but they didn't smile back. God knows, I had done some heinous things in my life . . . but enough for a doctor to joke about me dying? I thought I had come to terms with the bad things I had done but it was easy to forget that some people hadn't. I'm sure it had something to do with the massage parlor porn that was circulating around the world, starring me. Was that it? That's one of those things that's so outrageous. In the end, I can't be sure of any of it.

It was time for meds. I was convinced that the stuff they were giving me was destroying my mind, causing irreversible brain damage. The med was called Zyprexa and it made me feel flushed, indifferent, and hungry. I went from 160 to 175 pounds in my month in there. My plan was to trick the nurses into believing I was taking the pills when I would really be taking fake ones. All I would need is toilet paper and any fruit punch drink to mimic the color of the pill. I managed to make it pretty real at first glance. If you took a good look at it, forget it. I planned how I would act out the taking of the pill. I would have the fake one in my left hand, and after receiving the real one in my right, I would pocket it, then quickly swallow the fake one. It actually worked a few times, but the problem was that I'd have to keep making them at a regular pace. Twice a day. I was too lazy and depressed to stay alive.

My last memory of the hospitalization stay is about an escape plan. There were a good number of nurses and sometimes doctors there every day, which would make it difficult to break out. This wasn't going to be a half-assed attempt. It was all or nothing. There were security cameras all over the facility, including our individual rooms. Still, I was adamant about getting the hell out of there. There were two exit doors, one on either end of the hospital and both locked.

My plan was to wait by the door and pretend to be lost in thought, then when a nurse came through, I would catch the door with my foot, slip my shoe off, and have it act as a doorstop.

Finally, a doctor opened the door. I hesitated for a second, then took a dive, shoving my foot in the crack. I slipped out of my area into another compartment. There were some business offices as well as patient rooms. Was I free? There were at least ten people in and around but none of them seemed to notice I was there. I was carrying a book in my hand, as if I was a visitor and had brought it along to read. Blend in, I told myself.

At last, I came to the end of the corridor. Another set of locked doors. They opened suddenly. I could feel it was over. A couple of nurses stood there, shoulder to shoulder.

I politely said hello and began to move toward them, toward the open door.

"Excuse me," one said. "Aren't you a patient?"

I just stared at them. "I don't think so," was all I said. And that was that.

MERRY CHRISTMAS, UCLA

Mom

"The disease is a beast, an ever present, living night-mare that drives some to drink or drugs and even then, there is no escaping the torment that shadows them to the grave."

—Steve Lopez, columnist for the *Los Angeles Times*

Sitting on the edge of Jake's bed at Resnick Neuropsychiatric Hospital at UCLA on Christmas Eve with John, Molly, and my mom was utterly surreal. I think we all felt the seriousness of the previous month, and to have Jake spend most of December there was heartbreaking for us all.

There were daily visits and decisions to be made. I was told by a friend "in the know" to only put Jake's name on the paperwork, which made him the sole guarantor. He was unin-sured at the time. You know about that, the pre-existing con-ditions and all. The problem in these situations is that the family often goes down with the health care debt, and keeping it with Jake would allow him to file for bankruptcy down the line if needed. We couldn't help him if our credit was lost. These hospital stays rack up thousands a day. We just told them we'd figure it out and to please keep Jake there as long as it was necessary. The fear that he'd be released because we couldn't pay was unacceptable. We had already borrowed five thousand from John's work, just to get him settled there.

The nurses at UCLA were warm and informative. John and I could see that Jake was terrified and confused, but at least we knew without a doubt that this was the best place for him, especially following the nightmare at Alhambra. Dr. DeAntonio would come in each afternoon for five minutes. At first, I was angry that he didn't stay and talk to him more, so I called one night to express my concern. He told me that since Jake refused medication, he remained psychotic, and there was no point in trying to treat him in that condition. He was far too paranoid to connect with therapy.

At this point, with treatment not moving forward, the doctors suggested I allow the hospital to petition the court to order Jake to take his medication. A judge would come in to speak with him. A nurse being his support team would then take Jake to a room to meet with the judge. Jake, bless his heart, took this opportunity to plead his own case very seriously, not knowing the deck was already stacked against him. I was terrified to okay a process that would legally take away his right to refuse medication. I asked the doctor what would happen if he still refused? He told me they'd have to hold him down for the injection. I couldn't even imagine this. I felt sick.

"What would you do if this was your son," This was my go-to question if I trusted the doctor. He assured me he would indeed do this and that this was the only way. Jake could not go on this way. He was suffering and the illness was keeping him from understanding that he needed this medication to feel better. I couldn't imagine what this would do to him, forcing him to take something when he was already so terrified. I was assured that 90 percent of the time, patients acquiesced in lieu of anyone forcing something on them. He did indeed accept the pills.

It wasn't magic. These antipsychotics take some time to get into the system, and of course, we had to see if this was the one for him. I think, the first one they tried was Zyprexa (Olanzapine). There are also back up drugs to prevent seizures, which is a side effect from the antipsychotics.

It was a rough December. Bringing gifts for Jake to unwrap at Christmas seemed cruel. But not acknowledging it seemed unthinkable. What could he possibly want as a gift more than getting the hell out of there? We brought him a few brightly wrapped packages which stood out against the colorless backdrop of his room. He was depressed and there was little to lift his spirits. He was happy to see his grandma who was often his confidant and his kid sister, Molly, who stood by his side throughout, smiling and encouraging him, then sobbing on the elevator ride down to our car. It all seemed so unfair.

One afternoon, Becky and her husband sat with Jake in the center room, horrified at the situation, uncertain that he should even be in this place at all. Rehab for alcohol was one thing, but this was an altogether different beast, and during this highly stressful time, it created family friction coming from both sides. Well-meaning always. We were all scared.

One afternoon, Jake's dad and I brought him his favorite In and Out Burger meal with fries, in hopes that he'd brighten. For a moment, he smiled, then took a quick bite, but soon disappeared into his bathroom where we were certain he had spit it out. We quickly learned that his mistrust and fear of being harmed or poisoned extended to all people, even us, so we knew not to take it personally.

We visited every day, and I sometimes received calls from him at night from the payphone in the hall. These were unsettling conversations as nights were and still are his roughest time. Symptoms peak during these late hours. I know this as a worrier myself, that most people deal with all sorts of fears at bedtime. They seem bigger and scarier. Was that headache I had today a warning of something? I forgot to make the house payment, so I begin to visualize our bank account. Always worries about our children for various reasons are worse at night. Anyway, this tendency makes it easy to understand the worsening of mental illness symptoms after dark.

One afternoon, we were taken to a small conference room to talk with a few doctors and a nurse about the timing of Jake's release. They expressed concern about the rising hospital bill and our insurance situation. We begged them not to put that in the equation. We were already well beyond our ability to pay, so what was another five or ten thousand at this point! They were truly on our side, at least I thought so at the time. We wanted all they could offer our son.

Three days later, they released him, assuring us that with the medication they prescribed and continued therapy, he would be safe. We weren't so sure. Jake was happy but tentative on the drive home. He left with a diagnosis of major depression with psychosis. It was not going to go away, but now, it was time to help Jake find a way to live with it. But where to go? Whom to ask? This new road was well traveled but treacherous and dimly lit. Instinct, knowledge, and patience would be our guiding light.

HIGH SCHOOL AND PERSISTENCE
Mom

"Nothing in the world can take the place of persistence. Talent will not; nothing is more common than unsuccessful men with talent. Genius will not; unrewarded genius is almost a proverb. Education will not; the world is full of educated derelicts."

This quote by Calvin Coolidge hung inside the big bathroom in our house for many years. It became our family mantra.

About midway through Jake's sophomore year of high school, he came to us asking to go to a different school. He liked the kids and the place in general but felt that he didn't fit in. It was a very sport loving group, and most of the boys were into football, baseball, or both. He was so articulate in his desire to go elsewhere that we listened. He pitched his ideas like a lawyer until we set up a meeting with the school principal. She listened intently, then begged him to reconsider.

She told him she hated to let him go but could see that he'd thought it through, and that his mind was made up.

So, there we were, mid-year, without a school. We took him to a dozen places we'd looked up. All were small and each touted themselves as the answer for the creative or professional student that had lost their way. Promises were always made . . . most too good to be true. Jake's humor and determination got us through several more interviews. Each time, my husband and I were amazed at the quality of what we were finding available for kids who "fell through the cracks." I must say, there wasn't a hell of a lot of choice. Most are more than happy to sign you up and take your check but are pathetically lacking in the educational arena.

We finally settled on a small, impressive-looking school on a main street that was clean and modern and promised new laptops to each student upon acceptance. They also promised to get him integrated quickly and find his strengths. That was a joke . . . it wasn't cheap either, but we were desperate to get him settled and in good hands if that was possible.

Three weeks later, Jake still had no curriculum set, and of course, there were no laptops. They sidestepped that one very smoothly. The first day, a tall, gangly kid leaned over and said hello to Jake.

Jake smiled and said, "I just got accepted here."

The kid laughed. "Dude, they take anyone who pays. They don't give a shit about you."

Jake told us he was learning more about rebellion and where to get drugs. That was the end of that place.

Last stop on our search was a small school that seemed like the answer. There were a handful of students ranging in age from twelve to eighteen. A few of them were professional actors. By then, Jake had already missed a month of school. They too said they encouraged creativity and acknowledged his various learning issues. He needed structure, and I asked them to set up his classes for least anxiety. No algebra at this point, as I figured once he'd gotten things under his belt a bit more, then he could always go to the local valley college to pick up credits if he decided to go that way. As for now, I just wanted him to graduate from high school. He had a class there that was a sort of life prep—writing checks, balancing a checkbook, basic math, and other simple necessary tasks. It felt practical and yet we anguished at every step: *Where were we putting our son?* It all felt foreign and so risky, but what wasn't at this point?

In the end, this school was a hodgepodge of kids. One was most certainly bipolar and unmedicated at that, so there were many volatile episodes. Another boy was a sweet and fun pal, that is, until he told Jake his fantasy was to swing into the school on ropes and shoot it up like pirates. Jake was certain he was kidding. But was he?

Jake graduated in a class of three, so I tried to take charge of the all-school celebration which was a tentative twenty-five. I had to be sure that it wasn't a complete sham. We asked a dear family friend, Robert Picardo of *Star Trek* fame, to come in and give the graduation speech. We will forever be indebted to him as he was about the only thing that made that day special. He wrote and gave the most inspired speech. We'd later laugh at the backdrop of three students in cap and gown as the school director played "Pomp and Circumstance" on a tinny speaker at the Sportsman's Lodge in Studio City. Other parents seemed to have given up on fighting for a good school experience for their kids. It made me sad, this netherworld of lost children that didn't fit the mold of mainstream schooling. Why was that? Really, what about the ones who just don't fit? Or learned in a different way? What of them? Those days were filled with ominous foreshadowing of things to come.

LOOKING FOR JAKE

Jake

Valley Professional School was a very serious solution . . . at least, it was for me. I had been at Notre Dame High School for a year and a half. I was in the middle of my sophomore year and suddenly realized I didn't fit in. There were things that I liked there of course, like the Video Production Program and filming the School News, but mostly it left me feeling I was missing out on a real film education. I signed up for some classes at the American Film Institute, then petitioned my parents to leave ND and find a small school that would allow me the freedom to follow my dreams.

Leaving Notre Dame was scary, and after a month or so of searching for specialized schools, we found one that seemed perfect. On the surface, it was both friendly and serious for kids with "careers," but really it was just for kids who didn't fit anywhere else.

By the time I got to Valley Professional, I had tried out six or so specialty schools. I'd been told by one student that

Janet Jackson had gone there, and that her brother Michael was at her graduation in old lady hair and makeup.

The school's mantra was "Raw Talent," and they even had it imprinted on the side of their small building in North Hollywood. The teachers were as neurotic as the kids. Mr. Davis was a man-child who was obsessed with the deceased teen heartthrob Jonathon Brandis. Mr. Havorn was an overly sensitive math teacher with a hair-trigger temper. He punched out a student after being repeatedly bullied by the kid. There seemed to be no rules here. Not a good thing . . . but not entirely bad either.

I hardly said a word while attending good old VP and could've been mistaken for a mute. I was terrified of saying something stupid or offensive, which I'm realizing, as I write this, has become a leading obsessive thought in recent years. So, before this all began, pre-shitsophrenia . . . it was already percolating in my brain.

By the time I reached senior year, I would be thankful for the few girls my age that came to school each day. There was Katie and Claire Hawkes, a sisterly dream team who were all charm, good looks, and smarts. They could've made it as comedians or sketch comedy stars. They made me laugh constantly and feel comfortable enough to show them some of my videos, like the silly one of me doing chores, raking leaves outside. They looked at it, clapping their encouragement. "So, this is what you do after school . . . make movies?" Claire said, still grinning.

"Not all the time," I said back. "Most of the time" would have been the honest answer.

After school one day, the sisters invited me over to the apartment they lived in with their mom, then sat me down, and performed an interpretive dance to a pop song. It was hilarious. They were both brave and uninhibited, which is what I admired most, especially in Claire. I knew I liked her, more than a friend. I had never met anyone like her before. If I were able to take one thing out of my time at Valley Professional, it would've been my friendship with Claire.

During those couple of years, I shared a lot of my videos with that small group of appreciative classmates. Unlike Notre Dame High School where I'd been swallowed up by the masses, here for the first time, I had an identity. I was the funny movie guy. I decided I could live with that.

EXECUTED

Jake

It's usually at night when I get paranoid about something bad happening to me. On this particular night, I was convinced that someone was going to execute me in my sleep with a sniper rifle, or a SWAT team. Typically, SWAT teams bust down doors like the one that killed Osama bin Laden. Of course, the team assigned to kill me is empathetic. I don't know how I know that. I just know that they would have to quietly enter with their socks on and blow me away with a quick and accurate bullet to the head.

When I get this feeling, that the execution is about to happen, I check the Internet for clues. First, I visit Facebook because there has to be something about me on there. That night, the first thing I noticed was a new post by my friend Arne whom I've known for almost ten years from YouTube.

We have Karaoke tonight! He'd written it in bold print.

His friend responded, "Tonight?!?!"

Then Arne, "Yep."

His friend had said the word "tonight" with multiple exclamation and question marks. To me, this could only mean that "tonight" I was going to be executed. Shot in the head. That thought had been ingrained in my brain for so long.

About eight years ago, I remember being with my friends at a record store, and one of them made a random comment about a sniper rifle that seemed totally out of context in the situation. Boom!

A few years after that, my family and brother-in-law were having dinner at a restaurant. I watched him jump up to take his young son to the bathroom and when he came back to the table, he said he'd had a conversation with a sniper. Boom!

I wish I could go back to the beginning of when I first got this idea, but it's all too jumbled up in my head. This panic attack mode sends me to my mother with questions. "Is everything okay? I mean, am I safe tonight?"

She calmly looks at me in those moments, without hesitation or a doubt in her mind. "You are totally safe. I promise. Stay with logic. If you were in danger, I'd be freaking out too." After a few minutes, she convinces me to go on a walk with my sister Molly who always quiets my fears.

I haven't completely shaken off my paranoia on the walk. We talk about movies and different TV shows. There are so many. She mentions a documentary she watched, and I ask her about it. She seems reluctant to answer. "It's about some old guy who gets away with murder," she says. That sentence latched onto my brain and made me wonder. Was I a killer? Did I kill someone and couldn't remember it?

I am told that this is paranoia, but it's always in my life. I want to put these thoughts in a lockbox and pitch it off a cliff.

END OF THE LINE

Jake

My dad woke me up at 9:30 a.m. and I felt immediately depressed. What was I doing with my life? My parents are waking me up. I can't even get up on my own. Things must change. I feel exposed, eyes on me wherever I go. It's the circus of ME, 24/7. The good thing is I can change it at any time. At least I hope I can. I just need to write something and talk to someone, and maybe my course will change. It might be obvious change, but more likely it will be subtle. It's ripe for the picking. All I have to do is reach out and pluck it.

It's terrifying to ask someone . . . anyone for help. But they're there. As Mr. Rogers's mother told him, "Watch for the helpers." Asking for help is an art unto itself. Just look at the homeless holding their signs. Each one is different. Some desperate, some funny. Some paragraphs long and some only four words. Maybe I need a sign.

Yesterday I was in line at my local CVS Pharmacy, thinking about helpers . . . with a bottle of wine in my hand. Honestly,

I'd just wanted to grab it and get out of there. Get home, where I wouldn't feel shame. I scanned the room and noted a female security guard by the entrance. She was always the life of the party. Ready to have a chat with anyone who was willing. I usually made eye contact with her and said hello, but after weeks of buying liquor there, I made a beeline for the booze and tried not to look her way.

It was hard to miss this other girl who walked into the store yelling for the cashier's attention. "Is there any way I could get some perfume over here?" She was cute, a tad overweight with pink hair and cleavage meant for people to fantasize her naked. "Perfume!?" she shouted again.

I was trying to understand how perfume related to me. How was it for me? Walking in my direction was a man carrying a six-pack of beer. He approached too quickly, "Is this the end of the line?" he asked.

Was it the end of the line? For me? The end of my life? Of course, he'd said it, so it must be about me. How many people in the pharmacy were acting for me? And if they were, was it because they wanted to help? Perhaps they were there to berate me for their own pleasure. Either way, I could have asked any one of them for help, and they would probably be enthusiastic about it. Right? I wish I knew.

BATTLE WEARY
Mom

The previous month has been brutal for me, in that, I have far too often lost my perspective in this whole thing. I feel guilty complaining in any way about this journey. After all, I remind myself, this is Jake's journey, and I tend to operate on pure mother lioness instinct, but now and then, I run aground. My temper flares because he's sleeping in yet another morning after I made five attempts to get him going. He says, "Yes," and even sits up in bed, so I leave him to get myself ready for the day. After a while, I return to a locked door.

I temper my annoyance and knock firmly while keeping my voice calm. "Hey, kiddo, let's go. Open the door."

He cracks the door slightly. "I'm up," he murmurs. And so, I leave calling over my shoulder that he needs to be sure to wash his hair and put on clean clothes. I've been here before with him in the teen hygiene battle years ago, teaching him, molding him into what I hoped would be a responsible adult. And he eventually became all those things. He really did. *So*

133

why are we here again? I ask myself. My breathing is shallow, and I have that returning sense of powerlessness. It flares inside of me, and I want to get rid of it. There's no place for it here.

Fifteen minutes later, I return and he's asleep in his recliner chair, unshowered, dressed in rumpled clothes, and as yet, unmedicated for the day. I lose my composure completely as I have grown weary of this routine. It seems so unfair to me . . . to ME, and I want him to know that I won't stand for it. I expect more **from** him and **for** him. For a moment, it all seems to rest on his low bar of accountability, so I lecture him about how life can only get better if he pushes himself a bit more. Makes more effort. His hygiene, I tell him, is part of that. I rattle on as if this piece of information should once again be a profound and original thought for him, but he looks back at me with bewildered eyes that barely mask such intense sadness that I want to cry. I am reminded once again how much is out of his control. He is the victim here. I am too. Or am I? I realize then that I am only battle-weary from protecting him. He is the one that is suffering and must fight his way to clarity every single day . . . every moment.

"I'm sorry, Mom," he whispers and looks away. I instantly hate myself for my own weakness. Whatever I want for him, he wants it a thousand times more.

"I'm the one who's sorry," I tell him softly. "How did you sleep last night? Any panics? Was it hard to get to sleep?"

"Yeah," he murmurs again with his eyes averted. "I had a really bad panic this morning. Same. 5:00 a.m. or so."

The panics are almost always him waking out of a sound sleep with heart pounding and choking on extra saliva in his throat, which is a side effect from one of his medications. He feels he can't breathe and will die in seconds. A terrifying way to start anyone's day . . . and this happens almost every day.

He tells me that he woke up feeling sad this morning, as if he was under a dark cloud. This depression might lift after an hour or two, but if he can't shake it off, it tends to bleed into his day and night, sucking him back into that place I can never quite reach. I see him on the fringes, and his strength in fighting it is valiant. He fights and occasionally wins but then is faced with the very same thing moments later, as if his brain will not let him have even the tiniest of victories. I wish I could take this from him.

The previous month, he has had at least two psychotic episodes, and both were when he was trying to step out and be more social. It often seems to start when he reaches out of the box and tries to expand his world and make it better. With hands slapped into submission, he turns to sleep or alcohol to numb the onslaught of thoughts that loop in his head.

I will never just accept this beast that controls him because he is still inside there with all the knowledge, wit, love, and artistic gifts that continue to grow despite and because of his diagnosis.

DISNEYLAND
Jake

The happiest place on earth, or so I thought. I began thinking of taking a trip to Disneyland a week or so before I decided to go. It would be awesome. Soaking up Disney memorabilia and going on rides for two days straight. I bought a day pass online and made hotel reservations at the Disneyland Hotel. After what seemed like weeks, the big day arrived.

It was a sixty- to ninety-minute drive depending on traffic. I got there on a Monday and planned to leave Wednesday. My hotel room was beautiful with a fancy pillow on the bed that read "When You Wish Upon a Star." I couldn't wait to get inside the park, so I gathered up my things for the day, a backpack with jacket and a Gatorade bottle filled with wine to keep me centered. There's a monorail that runs alongside the hotel that takes you inside the bowels of the park to Tomorrowland.

I exited the train and promised myself I would try to usurp my paranoia by eating in a public place. Here I was, stepping into Disneyland, directly in front of a restaurant. I got in line for a burger and fries, then sat down during a Star Wars Light Saber Show while I ate my food and listened to the actors.

"You're not dead already?" Han Solo yelled to Darth Vader. There was huge laughter from the audience around me. I stopped eating and looked at my food. Was this a joke about me being able to survive poisoning? With that, I reached into my bag and pulled out my wine. Chugging from the Gatorade bottle, I turned around to see if anyone was watching me drink. Ten minutes into my Disney day and I was already paranoid.

I decided to cheer myself up by going to the wildly popular Indiana Jones ride. I got in the single rider's lane and zoomed past the long line of people. Did they recognize me? I was positive they did. I imagined what they were saying to each other. "What's the crazy guy doing here alone?" I tried not to make eye contact.

I finally got a seat on the Indiana Jones car and tried to prepare myself for the unknown. The first thing you see when the ride starts is three doors with huge Egyptian faces. Then a booming voice, "Do not stare into the eyes of the idol. That would be dangerous. Very dangerous." This immediately set me off thinking that I was going to die. At the end of the ride, I saw the iconic image of Indiana Jones swinging on a rope in front of a rolling boulder. My car stopped in front of the stone for an unusual amount of time. Just as this happened, a man behind me yelled "Jump! You're going to die!" This of course destroyed any chance of feeling good after the ride, and I fell into a paranoid spiral.

I left the park that day with a terrible feeling of dread and looked forward to retiring to my hotel room for more wine. I began drinking a new bottle around 6:00 p.m. Once I finished that, I opened another and finished it off by around 8:00 p.m. My plan was to go back to the park at 9:00 p.m. when there were fewer people around. By the time 9:00 p.m. rolled around, I was totally incapacitated and, if possible, more lost in my head. I couldn't handle Disneyland. The crowds. People warning me I was in danger. The fact that I was alone and recognizable. They all knew me. I wanted to get out of Anaheim completely. I gathered my things, not even aware that I was about to drink and drive. I had already gotten one DUI in my life, and if I were to get another, that would mean jail time. I walked down to the front desk with my leather bag and backpack, then checked out as fast as I could. Would this nightmare never end?

REQUIEM FOR FANTASYLAND
Mom

I'm not sure what time we lost track of Jake that day. His texts had stopped, and all I had was the ability to check his bank account to see if he'd used his ATM card anywhere other than Disneyland. Once it got dark and it appeared he'd checked out of the hotel, we began to worry. He wasn't answering his phone. About 9:00 p.m., I discovered he'd made a purchase at Gelson's Market near the Sherman Oaks 5 movie theaters. An old haunt of his. So at least he was on home turf. His dad and I began calling his phone. I left several messages for him that we were on our way and knew where he was. A necessary threat or two in order to connect with his logic, the little that there was at that moment. He finally answered, his ragged voice whispering answers to all we needed to know. I quickly urged him not to get back into his car. We were almost there. My God, he sounded bad.

And so the episode ended. He had driven home drunk. A good forty-five- to sixty-minute trip with a couple of bottles of wine in him, and he stood before us, leaning against his car with a small bottle of whiskey in hand. All I remember from that night is gratitude. I swear it. That's all I could feel. He hadn't hurt anyone with his car, and he'd come home alive. What more could we ask?

SACRAMENTO
Jake

Last summer, I went to Sacramento with my parents and sister Molly to see her fiancé John in a production of *Newsies* at the Sacramento Music Circus. It was a one-hour flight that offered its own challenges, so I kept in mind that my dad had spent several summers working there and had told me it was a beautiful place to visit, plus I really wanted to be there for my soon to be brother-in-law, Johnny-boy. He's a good man and he gets me. Once checked into our hotel, I soon realized that we'd have to go to a restaurant, seeing that there was nothing to eat where we were staying. That made sense.

"Old Sacramento" was inviting at first with a huge train station at the border of town and creaky boardwalks that lined the small streets along with candy stores and saloons. I was fine then, enjoying a corner of the city exploring shops and eating ice cream without paranoia. We soon found the restaurant where we'd made a reservation and decided to take a look inside. John met us there for a quick meal before his show.

It was warm and seemed harmless inside. A cute hostess showed us the menu, and we looked around. Nobody was looking at us. It was going to be okay, even though I knew I wasn't going to order any food, but on viewing our table and the people seated around the room, I had a sudden moment of dread. This was going to be bad.

We all sat down, and at first, the conversation was simple and easy to follow, then the waitress came to the table. Here was the moment of truth. Was I going to order something and seem mentally stable? Or would I remain silent and have my paranoia spill out?

She looked at me and smiled. "And what about you?" she asked and waited.

"I'll have a BLT," was all I said. So that was that. Even though I knew I wouldn't be eating, I'd ordered the BLT.

I began to hear only pieces of conversations filtering in from other tables. Only the ones that would service my paranoia.

"*Murder,*" one said.

"*He's just stupid . . .*" from another direction.

"*. . . going to die . . .*"

Finally, I heard "*. . . and the poison . . .*"

There I was, in total meltdown, not sure how to move or react to people talking to me. I only responded with a nod or smile but was unable to speak at all. By the time the BLT arrived, I was in bad shape. I whispered to my mom that I needed to step outside. My paranoia chased me from the restaurant like a specter.

The weather outside was hot and humid as hell and made it hard to navigate or focus. I spotted some shade on a curb and sat down, heart pounding in my ears. I lit a cigarette and smoked all of it, fast. I'm not sure how long I sat there, but by the time the family found me, I had completely unraveled. Memory tells me it was one of the worst panic attacks I'd ever experienced. Little did I know that there was more to come.

BEER BRAWL

Mom

I quickly learned that alcoholism is a different animal when it's combined with mental illness. But is it really? I arrived at that way of thinking in a purely defensive mode. My son isn't just drinking for sport, a bad break-up, or ordinary addiction that people on the street, in business offices, or local pubs are trapped in. He's not one of those people who merely enjoys drinking a bit too much until they are sucked into the abyss of "hitting bottom," or espousing weekly/daily AA meetings. My son's pain is real, it's . . . exquisite. The kind of inner pain that demands escape. It's about survival and quieting a wild beast inside one's head.

My sister and brother both battled years of addiction. I am forcing myself to look back on their pain, their loss of dignity, and their loss of all things that mattered to them. Their pain was real, and it was exquisite. It demanded escape, just like Jake.

In the airport a few days ago, Jake, his dad, and I missed a flight from Sacramento to Burbank, so we needed to kill two hours. Molly had stayed behind to see *Newsies* again and fly home with her boyfriend. We headed to one of those sit-down airport pop-ups for a quick bite to eat.

It had only been an overnight, trip but traveling the past year had become a challenge for Jake and seemed to trigger his worst fears. Anyway, he was back to eating packaged food, so I watched him walk over to another food stall that had mostly pre-wrapped salads. He brought it back to our table in the restaurant and slid into the booth beside me.

I felt him turn his head to glance at me. "Do you think I could have a beer," he asked, as simple as could be.

My brain did a hyper-speed rerun of his multiple times in rehab, the nights he drank a full bottle of Jack plus a bottle of wine to "quiet his brain," the night only a few months ago when he went to Disneyland on his own and had a full-blown panic with auditory hallucinations that drove him to drink two bottles of Disneyland wine to calm himself. My mind raced through the hours he . . . and we anguished over how to handle things so that his mental state didn't deteriorate further as the alcohol kept his medication from working.

Anyway, here I sat looking at my son who gazed back at me with such sincerity that I burst out laughing. "Are you kidding me???" I spluttered in a loud whisper.

For a moment, I think he didn't get it. I mean it really seemed that he wanted to know what I thought. The irony was threatening to blow the top of my head off. "You don't really need an answer, right? I mean . . . you know you can't . . . and why you can't?" Of course, he could do whatever he wants. He's an adult but we've established this bond, or maybe it's a lifeline that keeps him tethered to reality.

He shrugs and gives up. I figured if he asked me, then he already knew the answer. It was an odd moment. Later, he told me he knew I'd say no, but he just wanted to see what I'd say.

So, this is what's different. Like taking his medication, he is unable to see that there is a valid, continuing problem that will keep him from ever drinking again. He needs to reevaluate constantly. Real . . . or not real? Alcoholic or mentally ill?

I'm going to give this one over to alcohol. Yep. For my own peace of mind, I will submit to the power of the beast. All the corny, repeated AA phrases come back to me. They are true. Alcohol. We are powerless against it. HE is powerless against it.

God grant him the serenity to accept the things he cannot change, the courage to change the things he can, and the wisdom to know the difference.

A-MEN!

PROMISES AND THE EMO GIRL
Jake

The day I got to rehab, I was hungover beyond belief. I slept in the back of my dad's car as my parents took me to Promises, a high-end place that I'm sure they had to dig deep for. I had no idea what to anticipate other than thirty days of sobriety.

I heard my parents discussing me with the intake staff as I lay on a couch in their rec room. I didn't mind them talking for me this time; after all, I was still drunk from the night before. I think I remember begging them to bring me here, although I can't imagine it now.

After my mom and dad left, I was guided into my room where there were two single beds. I pulled out the sound machine from my bag and set it up on the bedside table. The button for rain was a familiar friend. I lay on my back staring at the ceiling.

An hour passed and I began to hear voices outside my door. It must've been dinnertime. I was terrified and didn't want to talk to anyone. I could've sworn I heard my name in the conversation so with eyes closed, I tried to ignore the door opening as my new roommate entered. He was a big guy, at least six feet and stocky. We didn't talk much that first day, but as time went on, I learned to trust him.

I fell in love with a girl in rehab. I met her during a group therapy session. My first impression of Haley was that she was a sensitive emo wallflower with a chip on her shoulder. There she was, seated across from me, curled in a ball, legs drawn up in her chair, while her pretty face stayed half hidden by crossed arms. It was my turn to speak to the group. I think I said, "I feel alien. Totally alone. Like white noise from a television."

That was the first time I heard her voice. She giggled from beneath her folded arms. Another woman from the group nudged her and she went silent.

By the end of the week at Promises, almost everyone seemed to be in fairly good spirits. I hadn't spoken much to anyone and was more like a defensive fly on the wall. I recall trying to process everything that had happened in my adolescence, all the while listening to the other patients express their every memory. That was the way it was in rehab. No stone left unturned, but you had to be willing to unload or you'd go thirty days in silence.

A few days in, we were doing a meditation hike at a Zen Garden somewhere. I was walking alongside Haley when it happened. All the emotions just poured out of me. I wept uncontrollably and had to sit on the ground. This breakdown cemented our bond. She watched me, making sure I was okay . . . offering me the sock off her foot to blow my nose. You don't get any closer than that.

Everything was better from that point on. After breaking down in front of a group of people, things tend to get easier in terms of expressing yourself. I had a few weeks of feeling pretty good just hanging out with Haley, going to groups and meetings. At one point, I told a friend I thought she would look good in a summer dress. Then a few days later, she would shed her punk look and walk into the group with a yellow summer dress. It sort of freaked me out at first. Either way, I loved her even more. That was a great moment in my life.

By the time we graduated the thirty-day thing, we moved into the Sober Living facility a few blocks away. Haley and I lived in a house with other addicts. I finally began feeling comfortable in my own skin. We would joke around about other people, Alcoholics Anonymous, and life in general. I wasn't ready to ask her out or make a move. Plus, I had a feeling that my moment to do it had passed with the day of the summer dress.

One night, I was in Haley's room and asked her if I could kiss her. She said she wasn't sure yet and needed some time to figure it out. She then admitted she was bi-sexual but didn't say whether she leaned toward men or women. I was sad that I had waited too long to make my move, but that was just the way it went. It was what it was.

While this was all happening, I had been seeing an assigned rehab psychiatrist about my anxiety and addiction to alcohol. He had prescribed me an anti-psychotic without really diagnosing anything other than anxiety. Sensing he was all over the place, I told him that I needed something to counteract the tiredness I felt from the meds he'd given me. I'm not sure what it was, but he told me it would give me a kick, so not to take too much or I would "go crazy." Writing this now I realize I was in shaky hands at best.

Feeling depressed about what felt to me like Haley's rejection, I decided I needed to do something to get her attention. I don't know, maybe something that would get everyone's attention. I would keep taking those pills until I was crazy . . . or dead. Whichever came first. I began popping them at around 6:00 p.m. I was alone in my car, calling and leaving her messages. She wasn't picking up her phone. This made my brain feel even more erratic and depressed, so I took a few more.

I locked myself in a restaurant bathroom, looked around, and took another. When I arrived back at my sober living house hopped up on whatever it was, I saw Haley and started ranting at 1000 mph. The thoughts in my head came spilling out. She looked concerned, but I couldn't process anything outside of my own head . . . so I continued on. To this day, I can't remember a word I said, except that I loved her. The intense moment was all too much, and I bolted. Nowhere in particular, I just ran into the night. I found myself on the street where the house manager was waiting for me. I was suddenly terrified. I threatened to get in my car and leave, but he said he would call the cops if I did. "Do you want to go to jail . . . because I swear, I'll call the cops," he spoke softly, apparently following some protocol to keep the situation from escalating.

My only option was going back for another thirty days. I didn't think I could handle that but being in no shape to argue, I gave up and he drove me back to rehab. That was the last time I would ever see Haley.

I returned and was called into the supervisor's office, still high from what I'd taken the night before. It was hard to keep my eyes open. Everything seemed funny to me. Ironic perhaps.

She was furious, the supervisor. "How could you do something so irresponsible? So stupid?" I didn't respond. I just sat there watching her. She was so angry. She didn't let me get a word in. I felt sick. "Well," she finally said, "I guess we can take you back. Just don't fuck up this time."

BABIES FOR SALE

Mom

We watched Jake park his car across the street from our house late one night. He sat there in the dark for some time, then his door opened. He slowly climbed out, bent over, and vomited on the street. His dad immediately went out to safely escort him inside. Little was said at first, and surprisingly, he came into the den where I sat. I'll never forget the moment because he smiled at me. When I say he smiled, it was not really a smile because only his mouth formed the shape. His eyes filled with tears and his forehead tightened with emotion. "I need help," he whispered.

I was instantly frightened and wrapped my arms tight around him. John and I took him to Promises Rehab Facility first thing the next morning. We struggled to come up with the required five-thousand-dollar deposit on such short notice, but somehow, we managed.

Legally, Jake was over twenty-one, so he had to sign the papers to be admitted. He was so depressed and hungover, barely speaking. We left him in their care and went back each week for family day, which was parent therapy in a group with your loved one. For me, it was a bashing by twelve-step psychologists who hit me repeatedly with enabling my son. I tried to explain that he had to take medication, which was not a lot at that time as compared to what he takes now. Anyway, we sat beside him in the large circle and endured all the stories and other parents' tears and guilt. I went home and slept for hours after these sessions. There was more going on than alcohol addiction. I knew this then but couldn't find the answers we needed. In this place, alcohol was the master, the only answer to all questions. Mental illness was never addressed, as at this point, they felt if he stopped drinking, his problems would be solved.

Once Jake finished his thirty days of sobriety, they convinced us to send him on to sober living for another thirty days. This made sense and we understood that it would give him a more solid base.

I found the psychiatrist that Promises assigned him to be a cold customer. He was a twelve-step follower which I do not at all condemn, as I believe, in most cases, it's a sound structure for recovery; however, this doctor was shockingly free with dispensing medication to a patient in this fragile state of recovery. He gave Jake addictive medication that he then took into the sober living facility. It did not go through another channel.

All I can tell you is that I heard nothing about any problems with a girl during his stay and most especially, the few days before he was to come home. Sixty days sober, or so we were told. The morning of his release, I received a call from

Promises letting me know that Jake had relapsed the night before. I was absolutely stunned. How had this happened when he was in their care for a staggering amount of money? There was much fumbling for the answer.

John and I drove to Santa Monica to see Jake and found him in the backyard of the house along with a dozen other patients relaxing under the shade of a big tree. It was a weekend so there were other parents. Jake sat slouched in a lawn chair, hair disheveled and eyes unfocused. An entirely different person than we'd seen only a few days before. He was despondent and wanting to leave with us.

There was a harried visit from the supervisor who'd quickly slung a stethoscope around her neck as she approached us. I was furious. Jake had overdosed on their watch and spent the night on a couch with only a young assistant in charge rather than been taken to a hospital to be checked out. He could have died.

I think we were too rattled by our son's mental state to worry about kicking the asses of a few pompous know-it-alls that worked there by day. There was no doubt they'd screwed up and they knew it; so for the moment, that was enough.

Jake still sat with his head lowered when a girl approached him from behind. She was pretty and petite but had that same lost look. She placed her delicate fingers on Jake's shoulders, then leaned close to whisper to him, but instead she looked up at us with a little smile. "Jake and I are going to have babies together," she said sweetly, ". . . then we're going to sell them." With that, she walked away. We were all silent. I looked back at Jake. He had that same strange smile.

CRAZY PILLS

Jake

I thought I was in love with Haley and when she didn't call me back that day, I just couldn't bear the thought of her not liking me. Oversimplification? Maybe, but that was my mindset back then. I feared everything and everyone. I think I wanted to go crazy, like that psychiatrist told me I would, if I took too many of those pills. It seemed it would be easier to live that way. Crazy and free from all of this.

Today, crazy is the last thing I'd wish for myself.

JACKSON POLLOCK INSPIRATION
Mom

About two years ago, Jake began finding comfort in painting. He's always loved museums, galleries, and art in general, but after our family trip to the south of France when he was about twenty-four, he became fascinated by Picasso, Matisse, and Chagall. We were staying in a small village called Beaulieu Sur Mer and had easy access to the train that got us quickly to Nice in a matter of minutes.

This pocket of time in France worked like magic for Jake. Something wonderful still happens if he is outside his usual environment, preferably far away where he feels no one knows him. He was on the razor's edge of his brewing troubles, but this trip held it all at bay. He was excited about seeing all the museums as well as being out on his own. He bought a dapper hat and rode the train fearlessly. For ten days, he lived his dream. He came back to us at night with wonderful stories of what he'd discovered. One day, Jake led all of us back to Musée Picasso in Antibes. I remember watching him walk briskly ahead with such pride at sharing it all with us.

That whole trip had been in the works for years. It was from the money we had saved for John's and my twenty-fifth wedding anniversary. My mom, sister Marilyn, and nephew Ryan all came along with John, me, Jake, Becky, Molly, and her friend Caitlin, so it was an unwieldy group, yet still a glorious trip filled with adventure, joy, and, of course, the angst of nine family members all together in one house.

I found it fascinating that Jake handled that trip better than anyone and made the most of the opportunity. I believe it was to be the last such trip for him for some years, with unlimited possibilities and freedom from his thoughts.

On returning home, John and I encouraged him to go to Aaron Brothers craft store and pick out a few canvases and a set of acrylics to start. We stocked him with supplies and gave him a place to paint. He did nothing but paint for the next few months.

I volunteer at the Getty Center in Los Angeles, so I was able to take Jake to a speaker event there in which actor Ed Harris and his wife Amy Madigan shared their experience filming the movie *Pollock*. Harris was effusive about his journey to understand Jackson Pollock's art as well as his unstable self-destructive side. Jake of course was an avid fan of all things Ed Harris, most especially *The Truman Show*.

Jake sparked to the whole thing, and soon, our small "art studio" was a rainbow of splatter color. I watched his talent grow. When you have an adult child who has experienced the loss of what he dreamed of since he was nine years old, you pretty much do anything you can to encourage him to find another direction. It made us all feel hopeful. Even if this wasn't THE thing, it opened him up and made him feel creative and useful.

Jake had always aspired to be a movie director, and it wasn't a small hobby; it was everything he lived and breathed. He drew us all into his world through his films. So now, perhaps this could be a crossover. He could find another channel to express himself.

After a few months of work, Jake had produced a good number of paintings in varying sizes. All were contemporary and dealt with color and texture. John and I suggested that he might like to get a booth at the Melrose Trading Post in Hollywood. It was a large marketplace filled with art, jewelry, furniture, and clothing. About $75 for a booth. It was something he could feel good about.

We secured the booth and proceeded with our new business strategy. The actual day at the market went well, and although we lacked the experience in the venue to request a better location for maximum viewing, it was still a great success. Jake's Auntie Mair flew in from Seattle and shared the spot bringing her own artwork. His sister Molly worked the booth with him while his other sister Becky came with her family to offer support as well as to purchase one of the prints. All in all, a successful and exhausting experience. Two years ago, he was still able to handle social interactions, as long as he took a lot of breaks.

My takeaway from this adventure is that it plunged him back into life in a way that spoke contribution and self-worth. Mental illness tends to dry up the spirit, so sometimes all you can see is the loss, so I like to suggest things that are a little beyond his reach but will safely ignite the old creative fires.

Several of his works hang in our office today in Studio City as well as a few that art lovers and friends bought and hung in their homes. I suppose a good idea would be to create a website to sell the prints that he made. An idea for a rainy day.

THE TRUMAN SHOW
Jake

Funny that my mom mentioned Ed Harris and *The Truman Show*. That film has had a profound effect on my life. When I first saw it, I reacted emotionally to it. It put its hooks in me and wouldn't let go—people faking their emotional lives with the titular Truman. As I look back on old video footage of myself and my friends, it becomes more obvious that these friends were acting out their relationships with me, rather than living them.

There was an old video of one of them holding up a picture of me and asking strangers if they had seen me around. The stranger replied, "Yeah, I've seen him at the YMCA," *which is a clear reference to me being gay.* I'm never certain who I am really, but that guy had to have known.

Then there was another picture of me holding a pay phone receiver while someone else narrated his perspective, ". . . I saw him ripping out the phone cord. I think he was pissed." *A stark indication that I was repressed . . .* which I was

160

at the time. Who could have known all these things except someone who had been watching me, as they did in the film, *The Truman Show. Reader, you must admit you're a part of it.*

SUSPICION

Mom

Just when I think it's under control again, I get a nagging feeling that Jake is drinking again. Most of the time, I do not directly blame him, rather I blame the alcohol. The booze, but it's his brain . . . the schizophrenia, insidiously twisting the facts in his head, as if to say: *It's okay to drink, it keeps you on track. Keeps the demons at bay. It quiets your brain and if you're very careful to keep it a secret, then no harm is done. After all, you're never certain about the meds working anyway, right?*

Jake and I are both here in the office to write today. We arrived in separate cars. I look over at his big desk with its brown metal legs and reclaimed wood body. His laptop is open in front of him, and he is slumped down in his oversized office chair. His head is back, and dark glasses cover his eyes. He is sound asleep. Now what would you think? Experience tells me that he drank last night.

Could it be a side effect from the slight increase of his mood stabilizer? Not likely, as he was on that for a month without incident; besides both his doctors say that this sleepy side effect would not just come and go. It would be constant.

The sleepiness and disconnect lingers throughout the morning, then seem to lift by late afternoon. Evenings are replaced by anxiety, then panic attacks resume.

I mentioned that I thought he was taking all his medication, so you might wonder why I question this. I'll tell you exactly how complex this puzzle is. When Jake drinks, his medication's effectiveness is diminished so that his symptoms return. Another little factoid is that cigarette smoking can also alter how the meds work in much the same way. He smokes more, therefore, his medication benefit decreases.

In any case, I've been watching Jake take his pills in the morning so I can be certain he's staying on track. If I whittle down the possibilities and throw in gut instinct, I believe I'm correct in assuming that he drank last night . . . and probably other nights since Sacramento.

I wish it didn't matter, but it's the whole ball game. I now have a twist in the story that I will send your way.

This chapter was written so I could confront Jake about his drinking. I just read him everything up to this point. As I said, we left the house at the same time, but I made a stop to pick up lunch for myself, then drove along Ventura Blvd. I spotted Jake a few blocks ahead turning left onto the street our office was on. I approached, looking for his car that is always parked at #24 in the lot behind the building, but I was surprised to see it wasn't there. I slowed and began to pull in. Instead, his car was across the lot alongside the big garbage bin. He stood there beside it smoking a cigarette. I thought this was odd but "oh well, what wasn't these days?" I backed out the driveway and parked down the street in an open spot.

By the time I walked back to the lot, his car was in its proper place, #24. I strode past and headed toward the office building . . . then stopped. Why had he pulled up to the bin? Of course. I walked back and glanced over the top. There it was, the empty bottle of Jack Daniels plus two empty wine bottles right on the edge of the bin where he'd been standing. So, you see, I couldn't just walk in after that and bust him. This was not about shaming him over his late-night drinking habits. I wanted Jake to hear and see it through our writing process. Besides if I admitted I saw him, it could easily backfire and launch his paranoia, that he was being watched. Truth is, it was an innocent discovery.

Anyone who is of the AA or NA world will cringe at this scenario. OMG, she's enabling him by making it her own problem to solve. Just kick him out! Send him off to rehab. Let him hit bottom. Go to Al-Anon and heal yourself.

No matter what my knee jerk reaction might be (and I promise you, I have them), this is where mental illness and alcoholism part ways. Yes, an alcoholic is an alcoholic, but there is no way I'd put my mentally ill adult kid out onto the street. He's virtually defenseless. His bottom is an abyss. Without medication and therapy, where would he be? I have only to remember him handcuffed by police that night outside his girlfriend's apartment, drunk, bleeding, unmedicated, and terrified. Or the night I rode in an ambulance beside him from UCLA to that godawful Alhambra Psychiatric Hospital.

These were not simply drunk nights. They were altered brain nights where choices were not just alcohol impaired but riddled with psychotic terror inside his head.

I am not writing this to get into an argument with AA, for that is an institution for which I have great respect, but twelve-step is not for everyone. Dual Diagnosis and its red herring trails between mental illness and addiction is a whole different book, and I will not tread those waters. Not today.

Now, back to Jake's reaction. To my surprise he admitted that he'd not taken the extra dose of his Topamax (the mood stabilizer) the past two days, so that left one day that he actually did take it. All of this and he still denied drinking. Damnit. I thought this gave him the easy way out. So, I had to tell him about the bin. I eased into it, reassuring him that I was not shaming him or spying on him. I explained what I had seen. He was quiet. I remained gentle yet told him that his dream of living on his own, in his own apartment, could never ever happen if he could not, A, stay on his meds, and B, stop drinking. It was that simple. I then asked him how he felt.

"Busted," he said and gave me a small grin, "but I get it." Still, he seemed a bit shaky.

In Jake's defense, when he is head-clear and well-medicated, he understands all of it. Every nuance. But one must always remember that a person with schizophrenia is forever struggling to find reality. What is real, what isn't. I cannot stress that enough.

I'll end this chapter with the reminder I gave Jake today. If he has been drinking for the past few weeks and occasionally skipping his meds but still managed to come into the office each day and share his deepest, darkest thoughts in this book, then imagine what he could do if he stayed the course. He's that smart, that sensitive, and that creatively gifted. Always remember the road you must travel to get home. Keep it simple. Keep it structured. Keep it true.

STREAM OF CONSCIOUSNESS SUPER BOWL

Jake

It's difficult to write today. My cursor keeps jumping parts of the page, highlighting, then deleting huge paragraphs. Hard to control a word processor. Like my brain. Hard to think of what to write. Yesterday I wrote about a scene from *Jaws* that was stuck in my head.

I walked into the courtyard of our office building and immediately saw my favorite dog, a corgi. I had that strange feeling that it wasn't real. That it was a hologram.

Look out for the elevators.

Ku Klux Klan members watching Netflix.

Signs of being gay. I would want to touch the glove all day. Signs of being gay. Not being able to think about being gay. Am I? Thoughts racing, trying to let it flow. Let it be. Why can't I just let it be? Super Bowl today. Starts at 3:30, along with holy guacamole and those crazy commercials. Keep trying not to get pissed off when my cursor jumps to a differ-ent part of the page. It just happened again. I can't get over the fact that my computer is the faulty one. My mother and I have identical laptops. I haven't done anything to provoke mine to act up. Why me? Fucking hell, why me? I'm feeling tired today. Logy, if that's what the spelling is. I'm suddenly not even sure that's a real word. It would be worth looking up in the dictionary. I'm going to save my work now. Matthew McConaughey is doing voiceover for both Carl's Jr. and Buick. What's up with that, Matthew? I guess when the film money dries up, he can always count on the residuals. There are multi-colored Post-Its assorted page markers on my desk. They seem so handy, yet I haven't found a use for them yet. I feel sorry for them. And sorry for me. My grandmother's lamp is in the office with us. It's one of my favorite things of hers. It's made of popsicle sticks and marbles. My grandmother (Kuku is what we called her) left all kinds of memorabilia behind before she passed. She left at least ten or more notebooks full of journal entries. Do I feel guilty about reading them? Not really. My mom began reading them first, so that diminishes my shame.

FREE THOUGHTS
Mom

I find Jake's "Stream of Consciousness" chapters terribly intimate. He's let you into his head on a day that he's vulnerable. When do any of us allow ourselves raw freedom, without judgement or borders? Schizophrenia is unbridled, disordered thought without logic or comfort. Yet within its folds, there seems to be equal parts terror, irony, maze-like confusion, memories, and intelligence. We just walked through the Metropolitan Museum of Art in NYC last week and Jake was mesmerized by the surrealist works. Of course, he was. Surrealism seeks to release the creative potential of the unconscious mind . . . as in the irrational juxtaposition of images. And there you have it.

STREAM OF CONSCIOUSNESS YAWN

Jake

Today is a spectacular fuck-up. I can't start a sentence without restarting or editing it. The whole point of stream of consciousness is to write without thinking. I began my day at nine when my parents woke me up. I couldn't face what the hours consisted of, which was, at best, to go to the office and write about my issues. So, I stayed in bed an hour, maybe two, then got up and shuffled my way to the shower where the air was freezing. I had a terrible night and can't really recall what I felt, but I will do the best I can. I knew my heart was going to stop so I got up and walked off the sensation. This usually worked, as the adrenalin restarted everything and got me going. By the time the sun rose, the feeling of panic had worn off and I could face my day.

My parents were planning a small dinner party with relatives later, and I wanted to get out of the house before anyone arrived. I got in my car and headed for the local Rite Aid where I could get some snacks and cigarettes. I headed up to the register where a lady with a light mustache rang me up. She took one look at me and yawned expressively. At this point, it didn't really bother me. The yawning thing had been happening for years.

I left the store and looked to my right. There was a woman trying to save money for a children's foundation. I would have helped but I didn't have any cash on me . . . then it was my turn to pass her. She looked up and gave me a blank stare. *She must really hate me,* I thought.

Yesterday, I daydreamed of traveling at 100 mph in a convertible. I was about to fall off a cliff. Somewhere nearby, people stood watching as if it were a blood sport. I wasn't scared though. I was curious. The car's hood jettisoned down, and the tires flew off the ground. It was totaled instantly.

I love writing when there is motivation behind it. When you are your best editor and best audience. When you feel like you have something to contribute to the world. I imagine or am convinced that right now, at this moment, someone is reading what I am writing. What I mean by that is that I feel someone is hacking into my computer. Watching me.

I went to therapy before going to the office and managed to stay awake on the drive there with my mom. I can't remember what we talked about, but it helped. Throughout the session, I felt so tired, like I was going to pass out. A little sad. I told Jackie that I'd prefer having my mom in there with us today. I needed to be able to tell her when I was feeling paranoid. As our time passed, I began to stray from thoughts of death and started to become a part of the hour. Upon leaving, Jackie led us out of the office. I could have sworn as I passed her, she said, "insane" . . . very quietly. This freaked me out for a minute or two, and then I realized I didn't mind if she thought I was insane. She was helping me.

Then it was just Mom and me again. Just us, as we walked out of the building. We made our way to the local hangout where we could either go to the bookstore or have lunch. I didn't want to eat because I knew I'd be poisoned. My mom kept pushing me to try. "It's not the place," she said. "It's the day." Which is such a simple and utterly true statement. "Same shit. Different day," is another gem. So, we made our way into a nice little brunch place where we got a chicken salad sandwich, and I made it through the entire lunch without panicking.

IT'S NOT THE PLACE, IT'S THE DAY.

STREAM OF CONSCIOUSNESS WAR ZONE

Jake

Am I observant of anything? It's one of those ridiculous thoughts I've had while being a poolside concierge at age twenty-seven in Hollywood, California, of all places. The so-called eye of a storm that is rippling chlorinated water, hollering ten-year-olds smacking water weenies, and needy bikini-clad girls asking me to rearrange their chaise lounges.

So, I ask again, am I observant of anything? Of course, I am. It just seems like none of it makes sense sometimes. When I simplify the noise and stimuli, it comes down to people relaxing and having a good time. What seems to me like a war zone . . . to everyone else is an escape. If I take it from the perspective that I'm simply helping people, then it makes me feel like a grade A humanitarian. Looking again, I'm not helping the sick or homeless, but well monied pool bunnies, so maybe that drops me to a B.

If honesty is what people want or respond to, give it to them in droves. Life is too short not to connect. Every person is different. Respond to the world as it is. Judging others is a product of fear for me. It simplifies someone, rather than having to get to know them.

STREAM OF CONSCIOUSNESS WALKING AWAY

Jake

Why did he walk away? After a long chat about relationships that went way beyond lines of sexual orientation, I felt a little uncomfortable. Blake made an excuse to walk away. Instead of me fleeing first, he left. Usually, I can talk to a person about almost anything. You know, be open about myself, and there is also a moment where I get uncomfortable and walk away. This time, someone else did it. I was the champion. So, what's the thing to take away from this? Don't analyze. Was it about me? About him? Everyone gets socially awkward.

I see white teeth. I hear sounds more threatening than they are. But it's all manageable. Things are beginning to move to the other side. The side of reason. Last night, I got about an hour of sleep. Got blown off by a friend today. My mind is tired but then reenergized by a sense of calm. I'm still here. I'm still alive . . . but the paranoia is still here. Always here. Less often with the guests at the spa where I worked at twenty-three but more with my coworkers.

I feel nonsensical about it, in a good way. Ebbing, flowing in no particular order. Easier to do and say what I want. People are chatty with me. I am more accepting of the banality and meaninglessness of it all. I am meaningless . . . but important to myself. A laughable notion that precedes a complete and inevitable death.

Here's a conversation I had with Vino, a coworker I really liked.

ME: I'm a fuck-up.

VINO: No, you're not. You're fine . . . you're a smart kid. You need to get out and travel.

ME: Really?

VINO: Yeah. See the world. So, you don't end up shooting someone. . . . And go get laid!!!

ME: How often? Soon?

VINO: Yes. Men need to fuck.

ME: Wow. I've never heard someone just say that.

VINO: Believe it.

Vino was a great guy.

STREAM OF CONSCIOUSNESS HAIRCUT CHALLENGE

Jake

Facet, faceted, multifaceted. Library. Dictionary. Get off yourself. Get over yourself. Believe in something, anything other than your own abilities. Get out from under the rock, that precious underbelly of your sleeping hide. Stop collecting Coke tabs. Get over it!!! You're having a hard time. We all know that. A lot of things that should be easy, are awkward for you. "Just dive in," as Paramore would say. "If I survive, I'll dive back in," into the pool filled with dirty smelly human beings. If I can do that, then I'll make a certificate for myself. Best nester. Best woolly mammoth cowlicks. Best behavior in a hair salon. The worst salons or barbershops are the ones that seem to require you to have a conversation. Or the people who work there are required to be nice as well as keep up a conversation. Why is that??? Why barbershops and not salons? Is it worth it to buy yourself silence? What a horrible prerequisite on a job application. You have to be sociable.

Went to my therapist at 12:30 and could barely keep my eyes open. Thankfully, I had my mom in the room for balance. By the time I walked into the office, I felt better about myself. It seems to help. Later, we found a hair place that looked like a salon and sports bar together. I could imagine myself as an actual sports fan, geeking out over the decor and sports channel TVs stuck on the side of the mirrors. Of course, I wasn't. Was I? But the slight kid vibe made me feel a bit safer. I was worried I'd get a face full of lethal chemicals inside the face towel before my shave. Ended up waving it off just before it hit my face. "No, thank you," I said politely.

STREAM OF CONSCIOUSNESS PARANOIA

Jake

It's almost impossible to write something of worth to match the schizophrenia that I feel. I can recount certain times of my life but where's the beef? Where is the knock-down, drag-out paranoia? I know how I feel on a certain day, and that notion is easier to write about than it is to pick out old stories from my life. I feel like every day is a challenge and that the same issues never leave. Like being paranoid. Like someone poisoning me. Or someone killing me in the night with a gun or syringe.

CANDLE
Jake

For a few weeks, I had been setting my alarm for 5:00 a.m. to disrupt my sleep cycle and hopefully prevent another incident. Old game, same fix. I woke up again several hours later, thankfully sans heart failure. There's nothing like fear of dying to keep you motivated.

My mom drove me to therapy after we'd had a few hours of productive writing at the office. For the past couple of years, it's been our routine to drive to Westlake each week to spend forty-five minutes with my cognitive behavioral therapist. What is that? It's basically learning strategies to change thought patterns and behaviors. It's always been a non-threatening approach that never fails to bring me relief. It's a positive therapy if you find the right person, and Jackie is all of that for me. Today would be different.

On this particular day, we arrived at her office and made our way into the building. I was feeling okay. We walked through the big lobby and opened her waiting room door. The first thing I noticed was the foreign scent of vanilla. Usually there was a strong new-carpet odor that I'd eventually gotten used to . . . but today, it was all about the vanilla. It immediately made me paranoid, and I sat down determined to get through the session without bailing. We were ten minutes early, so Mom and I ended up talking, or I guess mostly me listening to her talk. She encouraged me to be honest if I decided to go to my session alone. I assured her I would.

About ten minutes passed and out came Jackie, all smiles with her usual friendly demeanor. I followed her in, signaling my mom to follow today. I was too freaked out. The office reeked of vanilla. It made me want to jump out a window. A few weeks ago, I was given some incense which I loved and was always burning. Lately though, I had become suspicious of the gift and thought it had some kind of deadly chemical inside it. I struggled to focus on the moment and Jackie's soothing voice, but I couldn't get my mind off the strong scent. There was a huge candle behind her on the desk, double wick, burning with a vengeance. I couldn't take my eyes off it.

She explained that her office power had shut down so all she had was the candle. I glanced at my mom who seemed calm and relaxed, but then maybe she was in on the candle excuse too. I remember sitting up on the edge of the sofa, trying to listen to Jackie's voice. "How was your week? You and your dad had a weekend to yourselves, right?"

I'm going to bail . . . going to leave. The vanilla candle is filling up my lungs with toxic fumes. I'm dying. Now.

I stood up quickly. "I have to go to the bathroom." I looked down at my mom and she was surprised. "I'll call you later," I said to her.

"Call me later???" She was worried. She had that face. I bolted out of the room and headed toward the building's bathroom down the hall. I didn't really have to go there but needed an excuse to fend off the panic attack that was coming fast. I passed the bathroom and hurried to the building exit, feeling the cold grip of the door's handlebar as I walked outside. Finally, I was safe. Safe from the threat and safe from my mind.

TRIGGERS THAT FLICKER

Mom

There are days that start one way and end another. This particular day is a Thursday, but because I'd been out of town visiting family for four to five days, Jake opted for my company. We stopped at our office to do some writing first, then drove to see Jackie as I chatted away about our book, and he dozed on and off beside me. I was excited about this new connection he had with his writing. All too often I seek some form of assurance from him, needing to be certain he'll tell me if he goes to a dark place that he can't handle. "Not today," he tells me smiling. "I'm good," is all he says. He is clearly enjoying himself even though I notice he seems a bit too sleepy today.

I have what my best friend refers to as parental PTSD. Daylight takes me to a place of extreme hope and glorious victory over his illness. At the same time, I have that weird ache deep inside me that is ever present and guarding against anything and everything that might derail his life and mine. We seem fused that way, rather than bonded.

We arrive fifteen minutes early and walk into the building. Jackie's outer office is almost always empty. A good thing really. A small quiet area. Jake reached over and clicked the light switch under his doctor's name to let her know he was there. He turned to look at me and said softly, "I hope Jackie won't be annoyed with me today."

I looked at him. "She's never annoyed. Especially not with you. You okay?"

"Yeah." His eyes darted to the left of me. "You can come in with me if you want," he said.

Then the door opened, and Jackie came out smiling. She was always extremely welcoming. A safe place for Jake. We walked into the small office, and I noticed the dim light right away. She quickly explained that her desk lamp had burned out, so she had placed a small vanilla candle that flickered against the wall toward the back of her desk. There was a floor lamp in the corner by the couch, which must have had a pretty low wattage bulb as it cast a tiny glow around the printer/copier. A peaceful feel, but a little too dark, even for me.

She always explained anything that might seem different in the office to Jake. Occasionally, there was a knock on the wall from another office and she'd go out of her way to explain that it was building maintenance and that even though we could hear them at work, they were not able to hear anything from our side. I often thought she over protected, but still, it was nice. Perceived safety was imperative. We all smiled about the candle, and I even said something about Jake having candles in his room from time to time. He nodded. We moved on.

On this day, we discussed how it felt to write and the cathartic nature of what Jake was experiencing by putting his most personal thoughts on paper. Sometimes paranoid thoughts, going back in his head to scarier times where he would try to make sense of what had happened to him on a particular day. I glanced over at him. He looked so handsome in the flickering light. Vulnerable.

In what appeared to be a sudden move, he leaned forward, then slid to the front edge of the couch. I stopped mid-sentence. "Are you okay?"

I could see he was distressed. "Yeah. Um, I have to go to the bathroom." He rose to his feet and stopped by the side of my chair, looking down at me. "I'll call you," he whispered.

"Wait. Are you coming back?" I was suddenly alarmed.

"Yeah." Then again, "I'll call you." He quickly walked out.

Jackie was standing by then, immediately wondering what had triggered what appeared to be a panic attack. I was certain I'd pushed him too hard, suggesting we write this book. What was I thinking? This was a huge leap to get an office and encourage him to step out into an area that most certainly would leave him feeling raw and exposed.

My cellphone rang in my purse, and I jumped for it. It was Jake, speaking a bit faster than usual. "I'm just . . . really paranoid right now. I can't come back in there. It's not you or Jackie." He assured me he would be alright and hung up. So like him to protect, letting us know it wasn't anyone's fault.

I found him sitting on the curb in the parking lot in front of our car. Smoking. Clearly anxious but not as bad as I'd feared.

I asked if it was about our writing and apologized for talking about it too much.

He looked up at me, "Not at all. It was the candle, Mom. It freaked me out."

Jake gradually relaxed. He said it was all about walking into an altered room. The dim light and smell of vanilla set an eerie scene that he just couldn't shake. That experience would linger throughout his day much like a hangover after a night of booze. A candle? Really? Triggers are everywhere, and I realize again what he is up against.

STARTING OVER
Jake

I wish there was a way to start over, to look back on the timeline of my life and choose where to begin again. As I look back, there are so many mistakes that I wouldn't know where to start.

I can't go outside without knowing there are people watching me live my life. Learning about themselves as they observe me. Watching how I respond to complete transparency. Knowing what I write. Knowing what I think. I saw a girl across the street today, directly parallel to the office where I write. She was looking at her phone. I thought, *Is she using the app or program that tracks me so that people can follow me?*

I always thought I was a government experiment. Instead of putting me in jail, they would watch me. Watch me make mistakes and observe me to learn about future criminals like me. There is only one way to let it go and start living my life and that is to embrace the situation I'm in. To talk to people about it. Even if they denied it, I would still get it out in the open. People observing me probably see me as a metaphor for secrets and insecurities in their own lives. They are thankful for the example to follow. And for a moment, I am grateful.

MYSTERIOUS MUSINGS

Mom

All those movies. His love and passion for film since he was nine years old until today. Movies taught him life, story, perspective. They expanded his imagination and allowed him to pour his intelligence and art into each frame. His goals and his dreams knew no bounds. His bookshelves are lined with film biographies and literally hundreds and hundreds of DVDs. He breathes each one: cinematography, directing, dialogue, and score.

Now his mind will at times get caught in a loop from those years that defined his childhood and formed his art. It tells him he is not safe, and that he lives in a world that has caged, watched, and betrayed him. Damn *The Truman Show*. Within that world beats the heart of schizophrenia.

RAINY DAY THOUGHTS
Mom

Today started out to be one of those flat, discouraged, and sad kind of days. Yeah, I get them too. Parents are so busy being tuned into their child and his or her problems that we forget to take care of ourselves. I must remind myself that it's okay to be tired. It's okay to be angry. It's okay to be crushed by the weight of it all and to want to just scream in your pillow.

In those moments, my anger at Jake not taking a medication or drinking the night before, right after we've spent two long sessions with his therapist working on the profound importance of his sobriety, hits me squarely in the gut. I instantly feel stupid that I didn't see it. Careless that I didn't catch it before it happened. I ache inside that I let myself believe it could be so easy. He's cured. His life will be good now and he can experience all the good things he so deserves.

I know better. When the pain is too much for me, I get angry . . . first at Jake, but that is quickly diluted because I know he can't help what's happening to him and he'd change it in a heartbeat if he could. So, within minutes I take a breath, walk away, and re-position my anger to go toe-to-toe with the illness itself. The fucking illness. Schizophrenia. I hate it so much. I'm trying to use the word more lately, so that it loses its power to shock. I hate how some of my friends go silent when the topic comes up. I realize they don't know what to say. I'm pretty sure they're a little bit afraid. After all, schizophrenia has nothing but bad press.

I find most of the "loved ones" coming to NAMI support groups have an adult child living at home, on the streets, or even in jail, and their tales, like ours, a mix of love and despair. A beloved child who seems to have fallen or dropped off the map with no warning. What would happen if we parents turned our backs on our mentally ill kids? Have you thought of that? Especially when they are in their twenties when most of this begins. It's called the prodromal phase. What the hell is wrong with him/her? She's acting weird. Saying outrageous things that make no sense. Maybe drinking too much and staying out all night. Drugs? Yeah, that too. Have they gotten a DUI? That first time is a doozy for all of us. You go to your mailbox one morning to find it stuffed full of ads and promotions from every tacky lawyer in town promising to get you out of the charges. A disgusting web of low life for the most part.

Let's say we kicked the kid out of the house because this was the last straw . . . a normal response, but by the time Jake got a DUI, I could see he wasn't truly aware of this new threat . . . just that drinking made his head quiet for a few hours. No scary thoughts. No voices. Racing paranoia was dimmed to a tolerable level. This wasn't a party high by any means. It was sheer relief. How could he ask for help when it was virtually impossible to put it into words. How could he speak of these bizarre symptoms that made no sense to another person.

I will address this to the parents who do not want to believe that there could be anything wrong with your child. He's just a partier, you say. A normal kid. Somewhere in there, you know in your gut that something is wrong. You do. Even though you aren't certain yet what it might be. It's insidious and is disguised with the sweet face of your child. Maybe they made a mistake because there is no way my kid could ever be one of those . . . mentally ill people.

Every time a person with schizophrenia has "an episode" . . . is psychotic, paranoid, confused, it does a little damage to a part of their brain. It makes it harder to return to that home base. Your child is trying to find his way home, so you need to wake up and recognize the signs.

Getting them on proper medication as soon as possible will take time and research. One of the hallmarks of this chronic brain disorder is that the person does not have the ability to recognize their own illness. Lack of insight. This is called anosognosia. Jake hates words like that. It's such a vague symptom, but it persists in a subtle way even after they are taking medication regularly.

These are critical early years when your job is to find a doctor or team of doctors that you trust. Call NAMI (National Alliance for Mental Illness), go to a support group, get suggestions and names. Educate yourself. Remember, schizophrenia is a biological disease. You will end up being your family member's case worker. Don't forget that. No matter how many people step in over the years, you are the only one who knows your loved one 24/7. Not to say you will always know more than the doctors, but your information is valuable. Sometimes imperative, and if you have a doctor who doesn't want your involvement, **then move on**. We love Jake's doctors, but it took years to settle into the right match. We all think of them as our team, and that's what you're going to need.

JAKE'S CHOICE

Mom

You were born. You were cared for. You certainly had a good childhood and all the opportunities that you wanted and needed. You had passion and drive for film from an early age. You created opportunities there and you dreamed big. Your imagination had no boundaries. Then something happened.

The twist in the road for you at around twenty-one came on suddenly and changed all the rules. It threw you to the ground, and with all the noise going on in your head, it filled you with fear, uncertainty, and unanswered questions. You grabbed onto alcohol as a Band-Aid. No surprise there. I'd do the same if I found the one and only answer to quiet the terror inside my head. Alcohol. I swear I would.

Pinocchio was lured away too, drawn to a magical place that looked so freeing and joyous. It was there he met the evil Stromboli who threw him in a cage and walked away with the key. Who has your key, Jake? You think your choices are gone and all you have left is the secret of alcohol that appears to work better than your meds. For a few hours, you can breathe easy; your problems are quieted or at least delayed. But they're still there. Open the cage!

The problem with drinking is the trade-off. You think you gave away all your free choice. The alcohol you chose has damaged your ability to take advantage of the good medicine your doctors have given you, and the booze totally guts the Clozapine's power to stop your paranoia and multiple fears. They grow. They thrive in that atmosphere.

In this world of hungover reality, you cannot move forward, though I do believe you want to. Mornings are impossible to navigate, afternoons are a cloud of Buspar, and evenings move into paranoia. If you drink enough days in a row, then your head will tell you those pills are not really that good anyway, that in fact, they could be hurting you. IT will tell you drinking is the only answer. IT will convince you to skip pills here and there. You will lie to people you love so you can stay in this netherworld.

I want to tell you that you do have a choice. You must feel good about yourself again. Want to accomplish the things that bring you joy so you can be close to those you love. **Then do it. This is your choice. Only your choice, and it's not tomorrow or next week. It's today. It's now. This moment.**

Stay out of the shadows and walk into the light . . . every day. For it is in the light that you will heal and grow. This will be the hardest thing you ever do.

So, kick the shit out of this thing and throw it off the cliffs of schizophrenia. Then let the wind blow through your hair and fill your lungs with freedom. And remember . . . I love you.

POISONOUS LOOP AND THE MAXIMUM DRUNK

Jake

It takes a lot of energy to hide liquor bottles from someone. First, there is pre-consumption, then there is post-consumption. At times, I hide them underneath my mattress. Or in my closet or in the pocket of a jacket. First here. Then there. Hard to imagine having this hide-and-seek problem at my age, but there are obvious complications that go along with this illness. Living at home with one's parents is number one.

Recently, my mother caught me in the act of dumping my booze bottles but approached the topic in a sideways manner. She simply asked me if I had been drinking at all lately. I said, "No," lying my ass off. Of course, she'd seen me, so the jig was up. I'd been drinking for some time by then. A few weeks, maybe more. She assured me she didn't want to send me to rehab again. So, I sit here at a crossroads. I can continue drinking or stop altogether. Or at least that's what I think.

I need more than anything to know that I have a bottle of wine somewhere, for when the house is quiet and there is no one left awake that can talk me through my terrors. I need the satisfaction that I'll be drunk later, my brain mercifully at peace for a brief time. Buying wine during the day takes away 50 percent of my anxiety before the drinking starts. It's the nighttime that's the worst for me.

Dinnertime can be perilous. Eating. My dad brought up his physical therapy session earlier in the day and how they used a body massage tool called a Theragun. "In the end," he said, "they just pound you into submission." He laughed then. I remember that.

What I heard was . . . the poison I consumed during the meal would be entering my bloodstream faster than usual. Hours later, that loop of paranoia was still active. That one comment by my dad had shifted me out of a logical mind and over to pure emotion. I was tuned into anything that sounded suspicious. During these times, I usually turn to my mom. She can talk me off the ledge every time. Thank God for that.

Sadly, that conversation wouldn't deter me from drinking that night. Once I felt safe, in the privacy of my room, I opened a bottle of wine and took a big slug. About thirty minutes later, I'd finished it. I'd tried to take it slow . . . maybe enjoy it, but I needed to get the maximum drunk, which is achievable either way, fast or slow, but the objective was to stop the relentless noise in my head.

I want to help my mom more than anything. By quitting drinking? Taking my meds on time? Sometimes, it's all damn near impossible but I'm getting closer to it. Tonight, I'll go online to an AA meeting chat room, and it will help marginally. I'm always afraid someone will know who I am, so I can't speak. So . . . the next meeting, I'll try again.

ZERO CREDIBILITY AND THE WEED
Mom

I've discovered a pitfall in my caregiver role these past few years with Jake. At times, my actions can lack common sense, pushing me into a behavior that is slightly irrational like the shenanigans regarding the weed I found in his room one afternoon. I was doing a walk through looking for my keys . . . okay, so I wasn't looking for my keys. I noticed a small ziplock bag on the floor and picked it up. Two large fruit flavored Tums, tucked into a small nest of what looked like dried grass. Grass??? Pot? It couldn't be. This wasn't his thing, and as I recalled, he went through a brief stage of smoking it years ago, then ended up hating the paranoid buzz it gave him. I looked back at the bag in my hand. Apparently, I was wrong.

I took a pinch of the dried substance from the bag and swept up one of the small lighters on the desk. I lit the end of it and surprisingly, it didn't burst into flames like I thought it would, rather just smoldered. I breathed it in. It was smoky, but there was a familiar scent. After all, I grew up in the 1960s, and my brother had been a long-haired, pot-smoking hippie for many years. I wondered if I was beginning to feel stoned. Anyway, I decided to take it in the house and share the news with his dad.

So, there we sat, John and I, side by side at his desk, hunched over the tiny bag of marijuana . . . lighting small bits and inhaling the smoke. We both wondered again if we might be getting high. Was my nonstop theorizing merely a *Mary Jane* fog?

The kitchen door down the hallway creaked open, signaling Jake's return from a trip to Target. I met him at the door, holding the bag up in front of him. He looked puzzled.

"I found your weed. How long have you been smoking?"

He didn't easily smile these days, but his grin was unmistakable. "Mom, that's not weed."

This wasn't going to be easy for him to admit. I kept my voice low and non-accusatory. I told him that Dad and I had lit it, and although it didn't have today's skunk scent, it had to be a different variety.

"It's not weed, I promise," he repeated dryly. "It's sunflower seeds."

I just wasn't ready to let it go. "It doesn't look like that. It's more like straw . . . dried grass."

His hands rested gently on my shoulders, and he sighed, the smile still lingering on his lips. "Mom, I chew them for the salt, then spit them out. That's what's left. I just hadn't thrown them away." He turned and left the room. A merciful choice, given that only now was I realizing we'd been lighting his soggy expelled sunflower seeds. I felt like an idiot. Talk about irrational behavior. So, let this be a warning to you about how far you take your suspicions.

The good thing was that it opened a casual avenue about addiction which was sorely in need of some lightness on all sides. It might seem bizarre to say it, but humor in the right place is . . . everything.

SINISTER BLOOD DRAW

Jake

I knew I had to give a blood sample at some point during the day, which had always freaked me out. Once a month like clockwork, I'd have to go to the clinic to do this or legally I couldn't get my medication, Clozapine. I was taking 300 mg a day at that point in time and they needed to monitor my white cells in case the number dropped too low. They say it's rare, but it can happen.

I arrived at the facility early on the staff's lunch break, so I just sat in my car for half an hour to wait for them to re-open. My dad texted me, asking if I was there. I couldn't text back because the clinic would be watching my texts. I knew they were becoming more afraid that I was coming in. "Oh, he's back," they'd be thinking, "the nice guy," I thought they said.

I recently figured out that people assumed I put on a fake personality because I didn't have one of my own. Was that a borderline personality trait? I lit a cigarette and tried to ignore my thoughts. Soon enough, their lunch break was over, and I headed up to the clinic. I approached the elevator at the same time as two cute Latino girls. Maybe they knew something about me and wanted to share it, but I didn't want to share their thoughts or the elevator with them, so I waited for the next one. Ding! There it was. An empty space for my pleasure.

I got off on floor three and found no one in the waiting room. Just me. Usually, I would think there might be a reason for this. Something sinister. Some kind of plot. Although I must admit even a room full of people would get me just as paranoid today. Hmm, once again it was not about the place but the day.

I waited for five minutes, and a cute phlebotomist in her twenties with braces grinned warmly and invited me into Room B. I sat down in a large leather-bound chair with a swiveling arm. She offered me paperwork, then sat down beside me. She was all business while she asked for various pieces of information. My heart rate increased a little when she grabbed the butterfly shaped syringe, but I relaxed into the ease of getting my blood drawn. I'd done it so many times now. I stared at the needle as it went into my arm. That used to send me into a cold panic. Not today. So, some things have gotten better. That gave me a moment of hope. I watched the blood flow into the small vial at the end. "That's it," she said.

I waited for her to press the ball of cotton over the blood spot, then put the elastic bandage safely in place. I turned and said, "Thank you" and she smiled again. Yes, today was a good day.

HEAVEN IS WHAT?

Mom

It was an unusually cool day in the early fall of 2019. Jake, John, and I piled into the car to go to a remarkable event in downtown Los Angeles called "We Rise" sponsored by the Los Angeles County Department of Mental Health, a large art exhibition relating to severe mental illness. This was our second year to attend. Jake had submitted three poems to the poetry contest and although he didn't win, they sent him an invitation to the event.

He wanted to see the 5:30 p.m. screening of a documentary called *Heaven Is a Traffic Jam on the 405*. There were panels on mental illness and a presentation on suicide in which the lead speaker was Mariel Hemingway. There were seven suicides in her family, including her famous grandfather Ernest Hemingway and her fashion model sister Margaux. Her sister Joan suffers from bipolar and schizophrenia. She spoke of "the pervasive stigma against depression-related issues."

Organizers and workers of this event were so quietly gracious and helpful that I found myself swallowing back tears. Jake was fully engaged. The art, the people, the hope. We all belonged here. These were people who got it. All of it.

We wandered room to room looking for the documentary film. Finally, we entered a rather small dark space with benches, a screen that was running some sort of art film, and beside the door we'd just come through, was a warmly lit popcorn machine just inviting us to dig in. A tall friendly woman told us the committee had changed the screening time from 5:30 to 8:30. She must have seen the disappointment in Jake's face because she immediately said, "You know what? I'll ask him to put it on for you right now." We sat on the benches and the movie began moments later. The film centers on artist Mindy Alper, whose remarkable art is now represented by top Los Angeles galleries. Her life is a balancing act of severe depression and fallout from her mental illness from a traumatic childhood. The medications she takes, many familiar to Jake, have not always contained her symptoms. Years ago, she chose electroshock therapy, which she credits for getting her life back but leaving her with a degree of brain damage. The film is about the power of creativity and an established LA artist Tom Wudl who has mentored Mindy for more than a decade.

We drove home exhausted but filled with hope. Jake was tremendously moved by this woman's struggle and the sheer brilliance of the art she produced during her time with Wudl. He had turned the darkness in her head into light that inspired. Who was this man who saw past her mental illness? And where was this amazing bright white studio from the documentary? I couldn't help but picture my son as a part of it.

I looked up the movie and found that it had won the Academy Award for Best Short Film the year before. Now, I was worried about contacting him. He was indeed in Los Angeles. A successful artist with work in galleries. He works with ten to twelve artists several times a week in a six-hour day at his studio downtown in the art district. Many of his students had master's degrees in fine arts, many with years of professional art experience behind them, and they had come to him as a master teacher. An art whisperer. I reminded myself, he'd also welcomed in Mindy, so in that was my greatest hope. I gave it my best shot by describing Jake's entire history, his painting, his creativity that had somehow gone dormant in a cloud of paranoia and medication. Cognitive therapy was beginning to bring some of it back, but he needed inspiration.

I wrote the email in a rush of feeling . . . then waited anxiously for a response. Surely, I would know something within a week. To my amazement, I received his answer an hour later. He understood my predicament but in fairness told me he had received similar letters "from people who see the film and write to me in a flush of excitement. Once that subsides or when it's time to actually mobilize the resources and initiate a process, I never hear from them again." He told me to think about it some more and so would he. We were to talk again in a week.

Hope can move very slowly. I was just a mom advocating for her son so I realized Tom Wudl would need to hear from Jake. Jake agreed with me and soon sent off an email telling Tom that he was "creatively bankrupt." He went on to share a little about himself, then pushed send. Tom called him within minutes, and they spoke briefly. An invitation to visit the studio followed. I was overwhelmed with the feeling that this was all meant to happen. You know that sense of being watched over by God, by loved ones who have passed, or was it just the magic of life? A plan unfolds. Yes, that must be it.

Jake joined one of Tom's classes the next week. It meant getting up and ready to walk out the door at 10:00 a.m. His medication was so sedating that it would be a rather large challenge, but he did it. I had to go back to his room seven or eight times to get him up, then sent with him a prepackaged lunch along with all meds necessary for the day. It was an hour's drive through Los Angeles traffic to the beautiful white studio, and he alternately slept and expressed his fears and "what ifs."

Dropping Jake in front of the building felt much like his first time at nursery school. He looked so young. He got out of the car with his equipment in a backpack; he turned to give me a long uncertain look. "Is this okay?" he whispered. Yes, yes, I told him brightly. He slowly walked to the door, looking back at one point with such vulnerability that I cried. Through this, I smiled broadly and thrust my thumbs up.

I picked him up five hours later. He came out smiling. He was full of energy. I easily saw his exhaustion, but it would be the first time in years that he had five hours without paranoia . . . or at least none he couldn't handle. This felt so hopeful. It still is, but there will always be bumps in the road. The days he wakes up too afraid to leave the house, those days are non-negotiable and clearly tell me he cannot handle it today.

But art offers him hope. A way to express the wordless, the silence, the terrors, and sometimes the glimmers of color in an all too often monochromatic world. I hang on to this every day.

ART IN TIMES OF COVID

Jake

I was excited yet terrified to join Tom Wudl's class. Was I a good enough artist? It turned out that it didn't matter if I was good. If you considered yourself an artist, you belonged in Tom's class.

At first, I was led to the back of the studio where Tom had set up a large piece of paper for me to paint. It was intimidating at first, but once I started to do shapes on the canvas, I relaxed a little. Before I knew it, twelve noon rolled around, and it was time for lunch break. Tom told me that I could join the rest of the class for lunch in the next room, but it was also perfectly fine for me to stay where I was until I got used to things. I took a deep breath knowing that if I didn't join the other students, I'd be thought of as a pariah or a non-joiner, so I collected myself and walked to the lunch area. I hadn't used the refrigerator because I was afraid someone would tamper with my food. Anyway, I'd brought a dry microwaveable meal. I sat down with it and tried to focus on the people closest to me. I asked the woman seated beside me, how she was doing. "How's your art going?" I asked.

"Oh, it's going well." She looked up and smiled warmly. "I'm making progress. How are you doing?"

She was so nice. I tried desperately to block out the other student voices and focus while I was talking to this woman, but their voices soon melded into negative thoughts. *He's never going to get out of here alive . . . He's crazy.*

By the time lunch ended, I finally managed to eat something, and my thoughts had quieted. I returned to my canvas, where I was alone, away from the other artists in the class. Later, I would join them again, but for now, I would be safe by myself. It was the perfect way to start. Work for an hour or so, then Tom would come around to me and offer suggestions. It was awesome. I had total artistic freedom and was encouraged by my classmates who would also comment on my work. The studio was stark white with splashes of color from the art by the students that surrounded me.

Over the next few months, I became almost completely comfortable in Tom's class. I moved from the back of the studio to the front where the other artists were. I made friends with two of the women there and got into a flow of conversation with them every time I went to class. I even became friends with Tom's assistant, Monica, who is a talented artist in her own right.

I found that though I was able to converse with people, it didn't mean it came without awkward moments. I felt sometimes I was saying something offensive or hurtful to the person I was talking to. Maybe evil. After a few minutes of chatting, it seemed like I had successfully reached the other side of a mountain without saying something awful. It was a detached feeling, talking without knowing what I was saying. But through it all, I'd made a connection. And that was something for me.

Then COVID-19 happened, and bit by bit, Los Angeles began to shut down until our studio's doors closed as well. It was a sad day.

ADRIFT ON A SEA OF UNCERTAINTY
COVID-19 AND CHAOS
Mom

It's so unfair. The wild card of 2020 was cast, and it changed everything. It will continue to alter our days for months and years to come. This week, the Capitol Building in Washington, D.C., was broken into by an angry mob. Another scene for our brains to digest along with images of our hospitals overflowing with COVID-19 and the bodies of lost souls stored in refrigerated bins in the parking lot. I couldn't sleep last night, which is happening all too often these days.

Now I want you to imagine what is happening in the minds of those burdened with mental illness, say someone with schizophrenia like Jake, who has recurring fears of dying and the gut-wrenching belief that the government knows what he's doing every minute. Not easy times when your delusions suddenly scream to life in a world gone pandemic-mad and the president of the country calls to arms a group of hair trigger white supremacists. The news is hard to stay away from these days, and John and I try to watch it when Jake is out of the house. There are a dozen triggers for his paranoia in one television show, let alone a news broadcast filled with toxicity.

I'm watching my son sink further into depression. A once-a-week FaceTime with his doctor isn't doing it. Once a month check in with his psychiatrist for meds adjustment is a joke. And here's the problem with all of this. A stand-alone topic for all of you to consider: **power struggles with your adult child and his psychiatric team.**

Any of you dealt with this one? God knows I have. Have you been denied information because your son/daughter has temporarily cut you from the loop? That's their legal right, no matter how bad things get for them.

We live with our son, manage his medication, give mental and emotional support, observe good days as well as the bad, and after years, I'm an expert on that. When Jake was four, I remember noticing that his eyes were a bit dull one day. He just didn't seem like himself. I took him to our pediatrician, Dr. Singer, who asked how I knew Jake was sick because there was no medical indication. I told him I just knew by looking at him. He told me he was getting used to trusting the mother's intuition and gave me a prescription to fill if Jake was sick in the next few days. Twenty-four hours later, he was running a temperature of 103. Ear infection.

And so, it is now, I look at his unfocused gaze, unsteady gait, and unwashed hair. I just know he's not doing well, that his symptoms are overwhelming him today.

I long for doctors like our pediatrician who gave weight to family knowledge and intuition. In the world of mental illness, it is harder to find these doctors who value that. Instead, there is fear of litigation. Fear that the patient might harm himself, and therefore, he is denied treatment. Yes, this happened to us. There is also judgement when you step forward to speak for your adult/child, who on most days cannot advocate clearly for himself. Instead, he might confuse what he's heard and what he fears. Where is the logic? What exactly is the real situation when he must take medication day after day and still feel that tomorrow might be "the day"? Who, if not the people that surround him 24/7, will have his back when talking to a doctor who sees him once a month for twenty to thirty minutes at most. I do. I have his back and I will not let go or be made to think that I'm controlling his life . . . even by him, because I know with all my heart that I only wish for his freedom from this nightmare illness. I long to see him take a deep breath and begin his day with joy, rediscover his editing career and the fire that was in his soul whenever he created a film. Then I dream of him finding a partner to share his life with and know that all choices ahead of him are his and his alone. These are things most parents take for granted: the day their sons and daughters learn to drive, go to college, get their first apartment, fall in love, get married, then create their own lives apart from you. This is the way it's supposed to be. I want that for my son. Schizophrenia has robbed him of that.

On that note, I will say that I believe he can have more. The Elyn Saks and John Nashes of the world aside, there must be more for him because I believe the quote that originated from Alexander Graham Bell, "When one door closes, another opens; but we often look so long and so regretfully upon the closed door that we do not see the one which has opened for us."

Stand strong, resist giving up or criticizing, as your child is still trapped inside his/her own head, fighting to get out. Reality, logic, and clarity will elude them at every turn, so it is our job to supply that without depleting our own reserve. Ay, there's the rub.

RIOTS AND COVID-19

Jake

Here I sit in the midst of the coronavirus crisis and George Floyd riots. Never so trapped. Never so isolated. Not only in my mind but very literally trapped. I've been in the outside world maybe ten times in over six months, but other than that, confined to my parents' house.

I wonder how much more social I would be without these events happening. What do I do normally? I go to the gas station for cigarettes. I go to CVS for liquor and snacks. Other than that, I hate to admit it, but that was the extent of my social life. I yearned to go to a bar or a club and swim with the fishes, but I never went. Now that there is a spotlight on all of us as a society and the choices we made to cause this pandemic, we are forced to judge what habits we had, as well as the people we spent time with.

I've been drinking a lot more since this all began last March. From weekly to nightly. I've progressed from wine to hard liquor. I can't say my paranoia has gotten worse, but its shape has changed. The riots have me wondering not only about my safety, but who among them is hacking into my computer. Am I offending the rioters? Are they going to hop our fence and strangle me in my bed?

LOSING GROUND
Mom

These are the days when my boy is literally hanging from the cliffs of schizophrenia. The loop of messages that repeat in his head, his brain a mass of white noise. It is impossible for him to focus on the life around him because there are grenades and minefields within him, and I fully connect to his isolation and fear. I know why he drinks, and I want to tell him it's okay because I have no faith in the medical community out there. But I don't say it, because I must stay on the side of logic and dare I say, hope. I'm the guardian of his body while his mind is at battle, which is today.

AMBIVALENCE

Jake

The virus creates fear and paranoia in me as much as the next Joe. Okay, probably more so. I wash my hands sometimes five times a day . . . counting as high as thirty. Do hopeless and angry people with the virus hatefully rub their hands over energy drinks at CVS before I buy them?

My rampant thoughts of people hacking into my computer and watching me from cameras mounted all over our house has gotten worse. I can't say why I feel more paranoid; maybe because I spend most of my time in this house where my fears take hold. I don't have any time off from these familiar walls.

I had a bad night recently, where I drank myself into near blackout, then rushed into my parents' room at 1:00 a.m. with all my worst terrors in a cloud around me. I was paranoid as hell. There is a threshold I pass every time I drink too much, and my meds cease working. It is living a recurrent nightmare, eyes wide open.

HOPE AND FAITH

Mom

For the past year and a half, time has hung heavy over us, yet oddly the months have flown by as there's not much on the calendar. For the most part, the pace of everyday life is nothing if not deliberate. There is something good in that for Jake. He's been sober five months by his own choice. No rehab. As John and I worked on our yard, planting vegetables in what we call our victory garden, we felt driven to make our property more secure by installing a gate across our driveway; the world news told us we'd be spending much more time at home in the future, so we made our own rules and gradually settled into some kind of routine. Routine. Structure. These are the building blocks that will cage in schizophrenia. The three of us talk openly now, and Jake finally expresses his paranoid thoughts and fears as they occur and is often able to stop them in their tracks. This isn't easy . . . but he tries and is rewarded each time. He has given his paranoia a name, **Bob**, which makes it a more tangible foe for all of us. A really good tool suggested by his doctor Jacquelyn, who is a godsend.

Anyway, there is light at the end of the road. Art class is back in session downtown, and although Jake is a bit out of practice socially, I can feel him stepping forward with much more strength. Schizophrenia is ever present, and the trick is to never let it get the upper hand.

It's funny that I find myself looking for a clean happy ending to our book, but there really is no such thing. Life isn't like that, especially on the days it's too complicated and heavy to bear. Quite often, there seems to be no one out there who can lighten this load. No website, book, hospital, or even doctor who gets the weight of it all. Doctors and psychiatrists are overwhelmed with the sheer number of mentally ill in need of answers. Most do not understand that the families often hold the key: the pain, the secrets, the inner workings of a mind with little logic to offer a clear road home.

There will never be a time that our Jake will be completely free from his symptoms, free from his deadly protective addictions that will seem like the only answer in those dark moments. This is acceptance.

"Some people cannot be cured, but everyone can heal."

GATHERED THOUGHTS
Jake

It's been over a year since I last wrote. Some things have changed for the better and some things have gotten worse. I'm taking more Haldol (antipsychotic) these days, which I think makes me function better socially, calmer, and more aware. I'm surprised everyday by this as I'm not usually a believer in meds and what they can achieve, but, in this case, they've actually helped.

As for the things that have gotten worse, I still can't shake the fear of the government coming after me, to shoot me in the head as I sleep.

The absolute permanence of schizophrenia is a nightmare. I can't imagine having to deal with it my entire life. I go to sleep with schizophrenia, and I wake up with schizophrenia. This is on a loop in my head, and I can't believe the power it has over me. It's taken years of my life for doctors to figure out the right combination of drugs to balance me, and that process is still ongoing. Many of my nights are terrifying and lonely, but those nights thankfully happen less often now.

On a good day, my hope is that I can speak to people from my heart and that I can see things as they really are. I long to love without fear and think with an unfiltered brain.

Logic rules! A simple statement I offer you as I wrap up this book. It will be hard to recognize and a battle to accept . . . but it will get you through the darkest places. The easiest solution for the most complicated problem: **logic**.

*www.jakemccook.com: This is a website to share Jake's artwork, video movies, and writing as well as a place to share your thoughts. Looking forward to hearing from you.

HELPFUL INFORMATION

www.JakeMccook.com is a website run by Jake. He shares his artwork, video and writing as well as offering you a place to share your thoughts and questions about *The Cliffs of Schizophrenia*.

National Alliance on Mental Illness (NAMI), nami.org:

NAMI is the nation's largest grassroots mental health organization. Find your local branch and join. There are many programs as well as support groups.

NAMI helpline can be reached Monday to Friday, 10:00 a.m. to 10:00 p.m. ET at 1-800-950-6264 or info@nami.org.

schizophrenia.com has loads of information as well as schizophrenia support and discussion forums.

DidiHirsch.org provides free mental health, substance use disorder, and suicide prevention. They also supply valuable information. This organization is in the Los Angeles area.

National Suicide Prevention Lifeline is a US-based suicide prevention network with over 160 crisis centers that provide 24/7 services on toll-free hotline: 1-800-273-8255 (TALK).

NIMH, or National Institute of Mental Health, is a lead federal agency for research on mental disorders: nimhinfo@nih.gov, 1-866-615-6464.

Brain and Behavior Research Foundation (bbrfoundation. org): Click on "schizophrenia" and you'll find a wealth of information on donations and current research. One hundred percent of every dollar donated for research is invested in their research grants: 646-681-4888/800-829-8289

Drinking Cons

Mom's Observations of Jake, before and after a Booze Night

In other words, *think* before you Drink.

- Brain zaps (that electrical current you feel in your head)
- Feeling of losing consciousness (part of early a.m. panic)
- Depression (feeling blue) and isolating
- Feelings of intense loneliness
- Strong paranoia
- Loss of reality
- Low sense of self-worth
- Lying to family and support system (doctors)
- Hiding bottles
- Inability to write or create with clarity
- Food fears increase (fear of being poisoned)
- Personal safety fears return
- Feeling of body shutting down and fears increase (sense of heart stopping)
- Risk of accidents or arrests if driving (fear of dying)

- Cross-talk returns

- Missed social opportunities

- Inability to go to movies that were once your "happy place"

- Inability to be social with your own family

- Message in your head: You CAN handle drinking. But you CAN'T!!!

Medication will NOT work when you drink! Medication is the ONLY thing that keeps all of the above items under control.

These are all the items on Jake's personal list. Others reading this may not have the exact same things and may have some that are not listed. Be sure to make your own list and hang it in your room where you will see it every day.

BIO

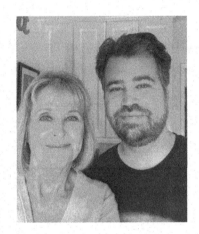

Jake McCook is an accomplished video editor and artist. He attended Los Angeles Film School Graduate Program, as well as Video Symphony's Avid Professional Program. He later won Best Editor of a Music Video, at the Elevate Film Festival, 2007. He currently studies art with Tom Wudl and last year his drawings were included in an exhibition in downtown Los Angeles.

Laurette McCook is a writer, and former actress. She recently completed a novel and hopes to publish it by the end of this year. She volunteers each week in the ER at Providence Tarzana Hospital, as well as at the Getty Center Museum in Los Angeles.

A TRIBUTE TO DR MARK DEANTONIO

Jake and I decided to contact Dr. Mark DeAntonio in the late summer of 2021 to ask him if he would write a quote for our book; after all, he was the psychiatrist who took the time to really understand Jake and was our guiding light through Jake's inpatient weeks at UCLA. I emailed him that August afternoon. As always he responded within a few hours. He'd read the material we sent him and he offered the quote below. We did not know he was sick and would be gone by December. We remain overwhelmed by the loss of a man who seemed to be the only person who truly 'got it'. I've gone back over my many DeAntonio emails. My lengthy and pithy laments filled with mother's terror and his brief but razor sharp replies that somehow in a few words, managed to hit the nail on the head every single time. Calmed me. Cared for my son. Brought reason to chaos. We will miss you, Mark DeAntonio with your motorcycle boots, contagious calm and brilliant mind.

"The Cliffs of Schizophrenia" is both therapeutic and meaningful. I worked with Jake at the beginning of his journey and was impressed with the love and caring he and his parents had for each other as well as their willingness to work collaboratively to challenge mental illness."

Dr. Mark DeAntonio, Professor of Clinical Psychiatry and Director of Inpatient Child/Adolescent Psychiatric at Resnick Neuropsychiatric Hospital at UCLA

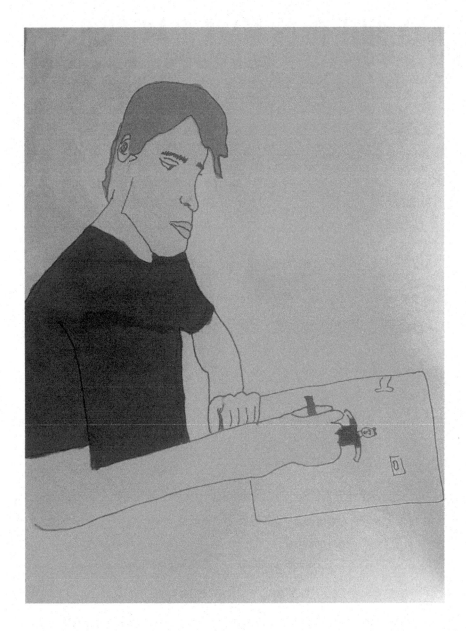

Art by Jake

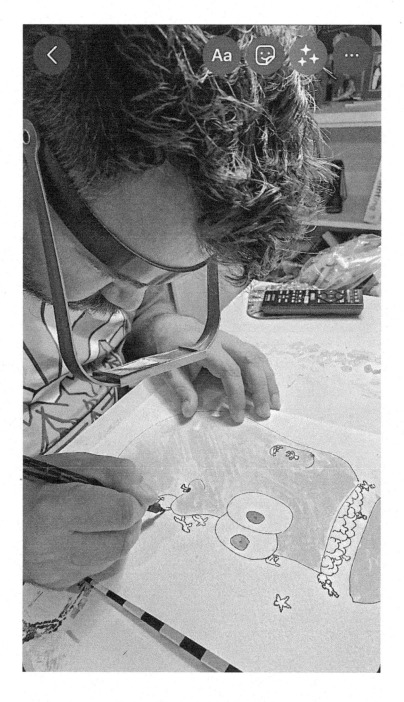

Jake at work in his studio

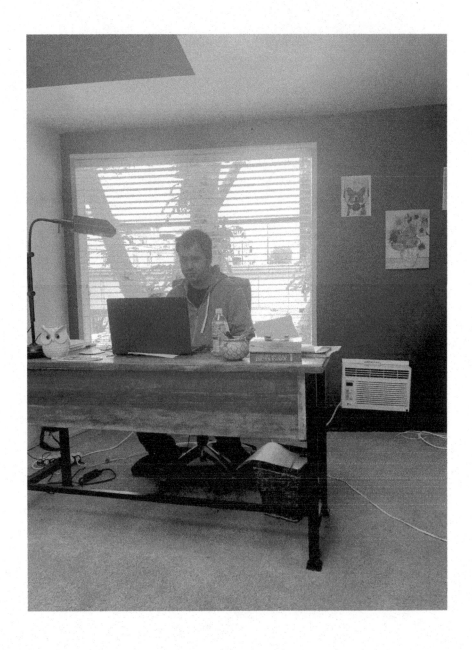

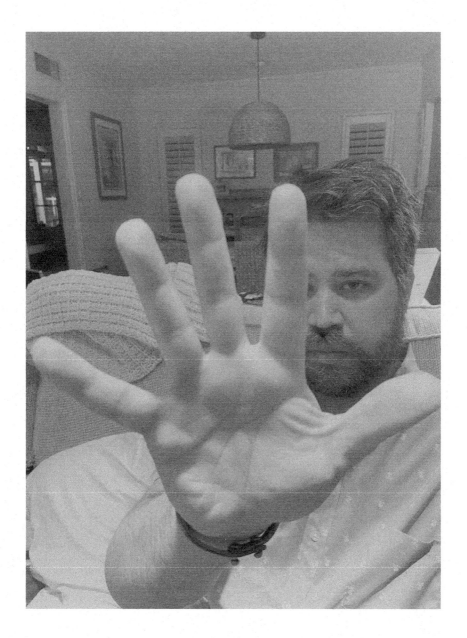

Stop

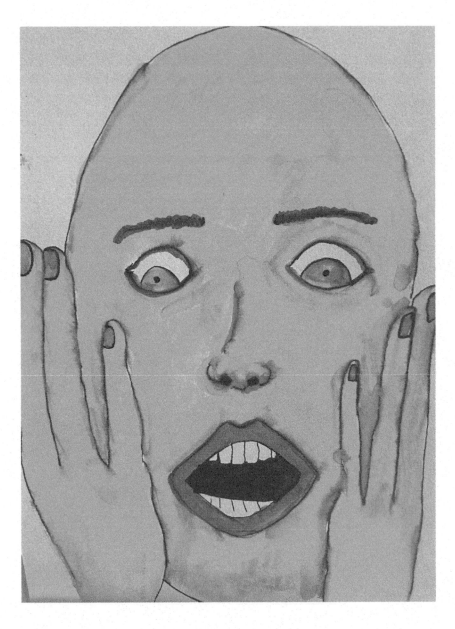

"Boom" Art by Jake

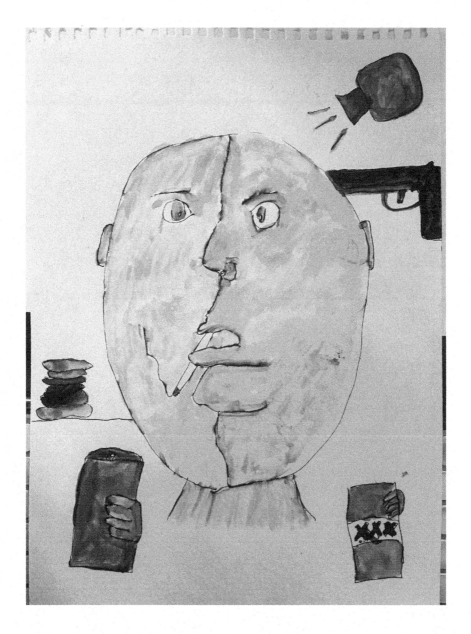

"Two-face" Art by Jake

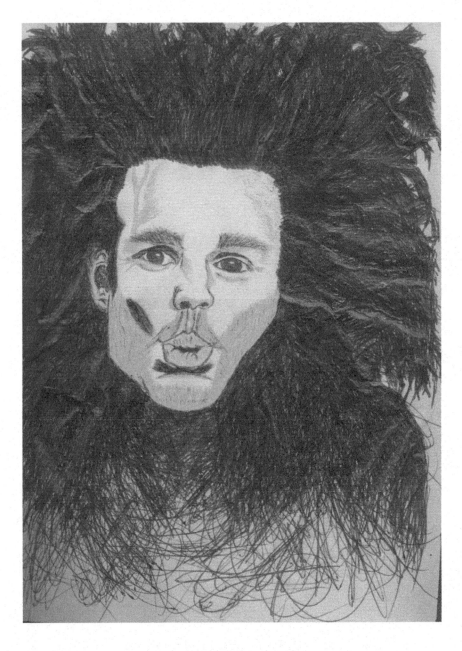

"Chaos" Art by Jake

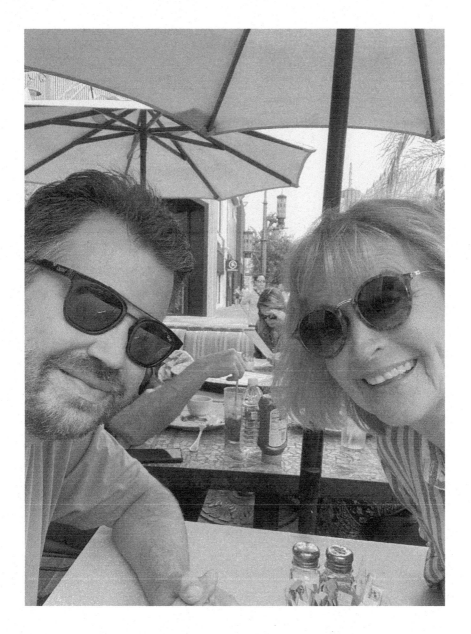

Laurette and Jake on a good day.